Marisa Peer studied hypnotherapy at th[e]
Institute of Los Angeles, known as the bes[t]
establishment in the world. She has spent [?]
ing with an extensive client list including royalty, rock stars,
actors, CEOs and professional and Olympic athletes. Marisa has
developed her own unique style, which is frequently referred to as
life-changing. Her previous book *You Can Be Thin* was published
in 2007.

Marisa works extensively on television and radio, appearing on
Supersize vs. Superskinny and *Celebrity Fit Club* UK and USA. In
May 2006, Marisa was named Best British Therapist by *Men's
Health* magazine and features in *Tatler*'s Guide to Britain's 250
Best Doctors. She gives lectures and workshops all over the world.

Visit her website at *www.marisapeer.com*

Praise for *You Can Be Thin*:

'The way Marisa Peer talked about the psychology of eating
struck a chord – and the effects were immediate. My attitude is
transformed'
Elle magazine

'Marisa is great. I've lost over a stone without even trying. I'd give
this nine out of ten'
Alexandra Heminsley, author of *Ex and the City*, on Radio 2's
The Weekender

'I'm always sceptical at the thought of another "miracle diet"
book but this really is different . . . constructive thoughts from a
woman who really does know'
You magazine

'I would recommend this book to my patients or anyone who wishes to change their weight and find a healthy relationship with food'
Dr Chris Steele, GP and resident doctor on *This Morning*

Praise for Marisa Peer:

'Marisa Peer has created a body of work that allows you to heal your old emotional wounds and feel great about yourself. There's nothing better than confidence and this book fills you with confidence. I highly recommend it'
Lynne Franks, businesswoman and author

'Marisa Peer has become internationally recognised for her profound insights in hypnotherapy. Her brilliance goes far beyond her early instinctive recognition. What has emerged is an incredible effectiveness, she is one of a few in history to have had a profound impact on the field of hypnotherapy. She has moulded the field of hypnotherapy into something much greater than it had ever been. Her latest work, *Ultimate Confidence*, is the latest evidence of her continuing evolution and profound knowledge in the people-helping professions. This book is a must for all practicing hypnotherapists and anyone seeking to transform their lives'
Gil Boyne, Director of the Hypnotism Training Institute

'Marisa Peer has an extraordinary skill at getting people to change. Since she worked with me my life has changed dramatically and for the better'
Jason Roberts, Premier League football player with Blackburn Rovers

'Every time I take on a new project in life, or face a particular challenge, I seek Marisa Peer's extraordinarily effective hypno-therapy. Marisa's therapeutic work and counsel is a hugely powerful

resource in my life, for which I am eternally grateful'
Gerry Cott, co-founder with Bob Geldof and ex-member
of The Boomtown Rats

'Marisa Peer is an absolute marvel. She not only changed my life, she actually saved it. Within two weeks of having just one session with her I stopped smoking and drinking for good and developed a completely different attitude to food. That was twenty-one years ago. I have never had a cigarette or drink since and I don't want or like unhealthy food anymore despite the fact that I used to devour too much of it.

At seventy-five I have so much vigour that astonishes others, which I directly attribute to Marisa. Because of Marisa Peer I have a whole new life. I cannot recommend her or her methods highly enough'
Molly Parkin, artist and writer

'Working with Marisa has really helped me to change some deep-rooted issues. I no longer use food to cope and I can finally visualize myself as slim. I am amazed at how much food I am leaving; I cannot finish food and I am indifferent to junk food, which is such a buzz for me. For the first time EVER I can work with food and it does not rule me at all'
Steven Wallis, chef and winner of *Masterchef* 2007

'Marisa's work is profoundly effective. She gets to the root of the food issue and liberates you from its vice like-grip'
Des'ree, singer

'Marisa helped me to eat differently'
Julie Goodyear, actress

'I had two sessions of hypnotherapy with Marisa Peer to lose some weight which I just could not seem to do alone. Within a matter of months I had lost over two stone; I have kept it off effortlessly for five years now. Marisa changed my life: her

programme works. I wholeheartedly recommend her book, it's worth buying it for the CD alone which is immensely helpful'
Mark Fuller, media personality, and CEO of Embassy Clubs and Concept Venues

'I know that without [Marisa's] help and guidance I would never have achieved my weight loss of over seven stone or been able to maintain it. What [Marisa] did for me is nothing short of miraculous. I owe [Marisa] my life'
Jeff Rudom, actor and ex-professional basketball player, participant in *Celebrity Fit Club* UK 2006

'Marisa is a gifted hypnotherapist whose methods work. I first worked with Marisa on *Celebrity Fit Club* in the UK. Her relaxed and professional approach meant that she struck up an easy rapport with the celebrities and she achieved results fast. One year later, I brought her to Los Angeles to film *Celebrity Fit Club* USA because we didn't find anyone in America as good as her. Again, her unique talents brought speedy and impressive results. She is unique in her weight-loss programme, I wholeheartedly recommend her to anyone wanting to achieve easy and sustainable weight loss. She will open your eyes and slim your body: her methods are brilliant'
Dagmar Charlton, producer of *Celebrity Fit Club* UK and USA

'I liked the way that [Marisa] changed the senses. As the saying goes, "people hate to be taught but they love to learn!"'
Phil Jesson, Director of Speaker Development, The Academy for Chief Executives

'I was inspired by [Marisa's] work and easy style and the way [Marisa] mixed facts with language with emotion with hypnosis, and how [she] worked on so many levels – very skilful – and beautifully executed'
Joanna Jesson, Chairman of The Academy for Chief Executives

ULTIMATE CONFIDENCE

The Secrets to Feeling Great About
Yourself Every Day

MARISA PEER

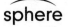

SPHERE

First published in Great Britain in 2009 by Sphere

7 9 10 8

Copyright © Marisa Peer 2009

The moral right of the author has been asserted.

A CIP catalogue record for this book
is available from the British Library.

ISBN 978-1-84744-138-6

Typeset in Sabon by M Rules
Printed and bound in Great Britain by
Clays Ltd, St Ives plc

Papers used by Sphere are from well-managed forests
and other responsible sources.

MIX
Paper from
responsible sources
FSC® C104740

Sphere
An imprint of
Little, Brown Book Group
Carmelite House
50 Victoria Embankment
London EC4Y 0DZ

An Hachette UK Company
www.hachette.co.uk

www.littlebrown.co.uk

Contents

To download the free hypnosis sessions which accompany the book please go to: www.marisapeer.com/ultimateconfidencedownload
Password: marisa

This book is dedicated to my lovely dad, Ron Peer, who always taught me that helping people is what life is all about.

And to all my family:
To my mum Dee, who is so supportive and loving. To Bree, Lucas, Carlyss and Isaac for so much unconditional love and for always filling me up with love and laughter. To Sian for being such a special and wonderful sister. To Cissie for everything. To my gorgeous Phaedra: my world is a better place every day because of you.

Very special thanks and acknowledgements to all my amazing friends, most especially Claudia Rosencrantz who has been the driving force in this book's existence by telling me for the last twelve years that I must write it. To Daniela Neumann, Helen Barbour, Jessica Richards, Charles Montagu, and Maria and Gordon Thomson: thank you for reading and re-reading my manuscripts, for supporting me, motivating me and most of all for believing in me and this book. I feel so blessed to have friends like you.

To my very own Peer group – Roy, Jez, Steve, Tim and Simon – who have inspired me, pushed me and supported me. Thank you for the Peer Pressure, it's so good.

To Eugenie Furniss for being an amazing agent. To Sarah Rustin for being the most extraordinary editor and for shaping and developing this book with me. To Rowan Lawton, Caroline Hogg, Kirsteen Astor and everyone at Little, Brown, huge thanks.

To Nicola Ibinson, Kate Taylor, Lily Hassan and everyone at First Artist Management, thank you for being fabulous. To Della for all her help. To Dr Susan Horsewood Lee for her ongoing and much appreciated support.

And to my own teachers, especially the remarkable Gil Boyne, none of this would exist if I had not been fortunate enough to meet you: you changed my life and I will never forget it.

'If one person breathes easier on the planet because of you, your life has a purpose.' And all of the above people do that for me all the time so thank you.

And finally a massive thank you to all my patients for your stories and for your kind permission to use them. This book could not exist without you. You have taught me as much as I ever taught you and I am so grateful for everything you have given me.

Foreword

I have known Marisa first professionally and then personally for over fifteen years and the day I met her was my lucky day. She is the most extraordinarily gifted therapist and I have sent her literally hundreds of people over the years, some international celebrities, some extremely famous, some a little bit famous and some not famous at all. They all had one thing in common: they needed help and I gave them her number knowing that she would change their life.

I can therefore easily say that her skills are unique and completely life-changing. Because of my high regard for her brilliant ability to change people's lives, and because of my job, I also gave her a significant role in one of my programmes, *Celebrity Fit Club*, where she worked with eight celebrities over a four month period and achieved extraordinary results. She is internationally considered to be the very best in her field and people travel from all over the world to seek her help. She is the only person I have ever met anywhere in the world who I know has the unique ability to help people with the widest assortment of problems, including those who have suffered the most severe forms of abuse, and achieve dramatic lifelong changes.

When people ask me why Marisa and her methods are different that's easy, here's what I say: when you have a heart problem, you go and talk to a heart specialist who diagnoses what is wrong and tells you that you need surgery. So you go and have surgery. If you just talked and talked to the heart specialist, that heart problem would be diagnosed but untreated and at best remain the same, at worst get a whole lot more serious. With Marisa, she is both the specialist who diagnoses and the surgeon who operates. You talk, but then you dive deep and sort it out.

I have been asking her to write her therapy book now for over twelve years, for all those people who just can't get to her or who she can't see. And here it is at last. And it is just wonderful. Full of her wit and wisdom. Full of her honesty and total lack of judgement. Full of her cutting-edge therapy.

For every single person who reads this book, it is their lucky day. Patterns and behaviour that make you unhappy do not need to stay that way for ever. People tend to accept that they are hopeless at this or that, they tell you that they have 'always' had relationships that go wrong, or do jobs they don't really enjoy – why?

Without even realising it, people adapt to their negative patterns until those patterns rule them. When you feel like that, or when your brain feels like Spaghetti Junction, just read this book and feel the knots unknot.

The brain can change and is happy to, if you help it develop new neural pathways. This book is just like a session with Marisa. It is effortless to read and to do, and then in the days and weeks that follow you just feel totally changed.

I hope every person who reads this book allows it to help them change their life. Marisa is wonderful and so is this book.

Claudia Rosencrantz, Director of Television, Virgin Media TV, former ITV Controller of Entertainment

ULTIMATE CONFIDENCE

INTRODUCTION

'Confidence comes not from always being right but from not fearing to be wrong' – Peter T. McIntyre

Why This Programme Works

There are so many books already published promising to show you how to be confident and promising instant results, but this book is different. This book reactivates the innate confidence you were born with and then massively increases it. This book takes you back to where and how your confidence became eroded and, through a series of simple exercises, regenerates within you lasting high self-confidence and high self-esteem. Within these pages are the keys to unlock everything that can and will give you lasting inner confidence and permanent self-esteem. Throughout this book I will focus on the methods that really achieve a lasting effect on your self-confidence. You are going to change your attitude, your language, your thinking, your beliefs and your whole mindset to become supremely confident and remain that way for good.

This book is written in a very specific hypnotic style using language patterns that will trigger significant changes in your thinking and in your mindset. It also includes an audio download link (see Contents page) that plays a very important role in reinforcing everything you have learnt in the book. Just reading the book and listening to the audio download will make you feel better about yourself and about what you are about to achieve.

The beauty of this book is that the repetition within it is designed to do all the work for you as you absorb the instructions and become fully receptive to change. That is why it is so worth your time to read it and do the exercises. You might just find it's the best investment you ever made. The hypnotic commands in this book don't require you to do what I say; it's not about following my advice or rules. Instead, the hypnosis triggers you to review what I say, absorb the information and then naturally implement changes, changes that are amazingly effective and permanent.

The method behind *Ultimate Confidence* is unique in that it offers you a way to regain the kind of quiet inner confidence that radiates out from you and makes an impression on the people around you. It shows you how to increase your sense of self-worth, self-esteem and self-value so that others will respond positively to you and even follow your lead and increase their sense of your worth and value. This is so much more than a book: it's a programme written to help you become the best you can be. It enables you to surpass your own expectations and those of others too, while motivating you to live your life to the fullest and achieve the things you really want with a new level of self-belief and with an inner confidence that will always be there. Through my approach to building confidence you are tapping into the vast reserves of confidence that we are all born with.

The programme's ten steps include exercises that free you from the past while giving you a more confident future. It has steps that you can use to improve your relationships, your career and your communication with anyone in any area of your life. It has case histories and client stories to learn from and includes proven habit breakers and psychological techniques that get results and can free you from anxiety and depression. It also has the secrets that successful people naturally use that you can implement into your daily life to permanently boost your confidence.

When addressing confidence it is worth distinguishing that it is not the same as motivation. There is a huge difference between someone telling you 'You can do it' and showing you 'You can do it' by giving you the specific tools and techniques that always work. Motivation does not always make us take action and it does not always come before action; often it is taking the action that then makes us motivated to do more. Sometimes when I go to the gym I am unmotivated and tell myself I will just do thirty minutes, and then I get into it and do sixty minutes or more as I start to enjoy it. Sometimes I am not motivated to write but as I begin it I get motivated to do more because I find the more I do the more highly motivated I become. Motivation means you can psyche yourself up to do something that may be challenging, such as going for an interview, or you can use motivation to make yourself take action. But when you are confident you don't need to constantly motivate yourself; you will feel sure that you can do things since, once you achieve real confidence, it's always with you.

The journey this book will take you on will subtly and irrevocably change your beliefs, your thoughts and your actions. You will learn specifically and in detail exactly how to visualise for success and discover for yourself the fact that scientists agree that visualisation can powerfully increase self-esteem. By the end of this book, when you come to A Day in the Life of the New, Confident You, you will be rewired to respond to any and every situation with more natural and easy confidence. You will have achieved so much and will be able to enjoy the success of liking yourself because, until you do, nothing really matters or has a real benefit. You will be rewired to be the person you were meant to be, and we are all meant to like ourselves. The definition of high self-esteem is actually how much you like yourself. You will be reprogrammed to have lasting, visible change in your self-esteem, self-confidence and your sense of self-worth.

The free audio download (see Contents page) is recorded as an exclusive session with me and it will help you keep all the changes you are going to make through reading *Ultimate Confidence*. The audio download is designed to reinforce everything this book will teach you so please don't play it until you have finished the book.

In my practice of over twenty years I have worked with thousands of clients who enjoy huge success, including supermodels, celebrities, millionaires and even royalty, yet they were not happy and did not have the self-esteem that you would expect given their achievements. I would be a millionaire too if I had a pound for all the times they told me they felt like fakes or frauds and were waiting for it to all go wrong, and that, despite seemingly having everything, they couldn't enjoy their lives because they lacked confidence and self-belief. I don't believe in instant confidence or the fake it till you make it concept; I have worked with so many clients who have faked it and have absolutely made it but still feel like they are faking it twenty years later and, as a result, they are unhappy, anxious and stressed and feel as if they are living a lie.

I always remember one of my very famous clients who had enjoyed fabulous success – including winning more than one Oscar – telling me that he was waiting for everyone to find out that it was just a fluke and he really had no talent at all. No amount of awards and gold statues on his mantelpiece alleviated his feeling of inadequacy because his inadequacy came from within. When people told him he was wonderful he didn't believe them and felt they had an agenda, or wanted something from him, or were bullshitters, or were so easily pleased that their opinion was worthless. His belief system had told him he was not good enough long ago and he had achieved fame to make everyone believe in him, but he still didn't believe in himself. This feeling of not being good enough is apparent in so many people, whether they're famous or not. Many people who have huge talent and have achieved success or fame are still very unhappy because they don't believe in themselves. This book will give you every technique that will allow you to believe in yourself, like yourself and feel good about yourself. You can't really have lasting confidence until you locate and remove the beliefs that make you doubt yourself; once you have done that you can have THE ultimate confidence – the kind of permanent, effortless confidence that becomes a part of who you are.

Many years ago I was reading a bestselling relationship book by a renowned author and was very taken with the chapter that said all you have to do to make a man feel great about himself is to praise him endlessly. Being a shrink myself I knew that was not strictly accurate. For praise to work it has to be intermittent and often unexpected and it has to be somewhat justified. Nevertheless, I tried this method with my boyfriend; he was someone who had issues with his self-worth, probably because he was dispatched to boarding school at seven. He was talented, successful, smart, very good looking and funny but did not believe in himself, so I decide to practise on him and praised him a lot and was rather surprised at his reaction: he became angry and irritable. I praised him for what he looked like and that produced irritation; so I praised his conversation skills but he didn't like that either; and later on in bed I praised his skills (and they were very good) and he just got more and more pissed off until finally he asked me what I wanted and why I kept on telling him stuff that he knew was not true. I really wanted to write to the author of that book and ask him what to do with his advice when the person you are praising won't let it in and won't believe a word you are saying. It sort of proved my point that when people feel they aren't good enough what you believe about them is less important than what they believe about themselves. You have to change your own habits of thought (your beliefs) before you can change your habits of confidence. This book will locate the beliefs that have been holding you back and then eliminate them for good.

How This Programme Is Different

This programme is different because it does not show you how to get yourself into a confident state by engaging in physical or mental exercise of the kind that athletes or performers use before a performance. Doing this is called 'getting into state' and the techniques to get you into a confident state do work but have to be repeated at every situation.

I want to give you an inner confidence that will always be there within you.

The major cause of lacking confidence is because at some level we don't feel good enough. Feeling not good enough is a horrible, pervasive feeling that we are always trying to compensate for by achieving more, working harder, looking better and getting better results. However, once you are free of this feeling and can know with unshakeable certainty that you are good enough, you will no longer need to battle with the feeling as it will no longer exist within you.

This feeling of not being good enough is something I've come across many times as a therapist to the stars in Britain and America. Over time I have developed certain techniques of my own that achieve amazing results. I've become known as a top therapist and have won awards, including being voted Britain's best therapist, for my methods. I've devised particular techniques that have become my favourites because they are so effective and many clients have written to me to tell me just how powerful and effective they found them. These techniques are all here in the book so you can benefit from them too. Having personally experienced low self-esteem and almost no confidence in the past, it always thrills me when I can instil the same great changes in others that I instilled in myself and my patients.

Like many people, I started off quite well. My parents were pleased with their little daughter and my grandmother always told me I was a genius. I even won a prize for being the smartest person in my year, but somewhere it all began to unravel and I became insecure, self-conscious and lacking in confidence. I also thought I was hideous to look at, too. I was tall and gangly from seven to about fifteen and thought I was supremely ugly, like a daddy-long-legs. The boys at school called me Twiglet because that's what my skinny legs and knobbly knees reminded them of. Eventually I grew into myself and at seventeen got a great boyfriend who loved my long limbs and thought I was wonderful, but because of my experience of growing up I always felt like I was acting, pretending to be confident, when inside I was a mass of insecurity. At one stage I was living in Los Angeles teaching aerobics for Jane Fonda and had a gorgeous fiancé, but the stress of pretending to be confident and self-assured was horrible. I always felt that because the way I felt about myself was so different from the way he saw me, it meant that he didn't really know me and loved a person who did not really exist. I felt that if he knew the real me he would be disappointed, so I put on an act of being confident 24/7, which was a huge mistake because, when people liked me, I felt like it was the act they liked and not the real me, which made me even more insecure. It's odd to look back at the person I was then because it seems as if who I was then was another person altogether. Having gone from feeling I was never enough to being more than happy with who I am, I want you to get the same results, and this book will give that to you.

My purpose for writing this book is to invite everyone who reads it to get back the confidence nature instilled in us and use it to have a happier, more fulfilled life. For years my clients have asked me to write out my methods and techniques because for the first time it is a way to achieve inner change that really makes sense to them and it works. This book will give you the same therapy and the same results from the privacy and comfort of your sofa in an effective and easy-to-follow approach. My patients swear by my methods to such an extent that I have never, ever had to advertise for clients; they have all come along by personal recommendation.

Why the Results Last

Following the processes in this book will allow you to change your habits of thought and then your habits of action so you make permanent emotional adjustments, ensuring you change from the inside as well as changing on the outside. The benefits to be gained from this book come from doing the exercises rather than just reading them. Do all the exercises in the sequence in which they are they are written and you will get great results. Really use this book by highlighting parts that you really relate to, using the techniques and exercises as they are written and recognising this is a process more than a book. Think of it as a journey to fantastic inner confidence and self-esteem. To get to your destination you need to complete the journey; if you get off early you will miss the best bit. The great thing about making mental changes is that it's free; it's instant, painless and easy. The adjustments and changes I will ask you to make are often small and simple but the benefits can be huge and life changing. When you are making physical changes there is no doubt that the harder you work the better the results will be. With mental changes the opposite applies. It does not require huge effort or constant and ongoing work, it just requires that you do it and spend a few moments every day reinforcing it in your mind.

You have a few moments every day, don't you?

Many of the mental changes I will introduce can be reinforced when you are lying in the bath, travelling to work, even when you are cleaning your teeth. Since you spend all day thinking and communicating with yourself you are going to continue doing that only so much more productively.

Everyone has a few minutes in their day.

This may be a hypnosis book but it isn't going to send you to sleep; it's going to wake you up.

The Benefits of Your Free Download

The session recorded on the free audio download (see Contents page for link) is powerful enough in itself to achieve results. However, I am a great believer in the saying 'You can't heal what you can't feel' or, in more simple terms, you can't fix what you don't understand. The book will take you through an understanding of how and why your confidence became diminished and show you how to reinstate it. The programme really gets to the root of any issues you may have that are affecting your confidence and builds from there, while listening to the audio download repeatedly for a few weeks will lock in all the new suggestions, building on the essential foundations that the programme lays until very quickly being confident is not something that you consciously work at, but is a permanent part of you. Listening to the audio download is like having a private session with me which will flood your mind with the images, words and beliefs that are necessary to achieving confidence and maintaining it permanently.

One of the rules of the mind is that it cannot hold conflicting thoughts or feel conflicting emotions, so while your mind is filled with confident thoughts and motivating images you cannot be thinking of or focusing on negative thoughts and images. For this reason this book is written in a style that makes changes to your thinking to ensure that this conflict of thoughts and beliefs ends, and the powerful audio download enhances those changes and permanently locks them into your mind so that you benefit from lasting, lifelong confidence. Every exercise you do in the book and every chapter you read will be compounded and enhanced by repeatedly listening to the audio download, so please be sure to wait until you have finished the book before you play the audio download.

STEP 1

'*The greatest discovery of my generation is that human beings can alter their lives by altering their attitudes of mind*' – William James (1842–1910), US psychologist

Attitude Adjustment to Get Results

It's useful to think of confidence as a journey. We come on to the planet loaded with confidence, only to lose a lot of it during adolescence; we then spend many years trying to get it back but not really sure how to. This programme will give you back all the confidence that is your birthright and the journey to get it back is simple and workable. As you change your attitude, your beliefs, your thoughts and your language you will dramatically increase your confidence.

Changing your attitude begins as something that you do and then it becomes who you are. I can hardly recognise the insecure, self-conscious person I once was. When I was working in Chicago some years ago I met up with my lovely ex-boyfriend from LA. I had not seen him for about ten years and when he asked me what I had done to change so much I said, I don't really know what I have done; it's not what I do it's who I am, and it's true. First I had to make myself change, I had to make myself do things that did not come naturally and eventually it stopped being what I did and became part of my behaviour and a part of me. I learnt specific methods of thinking and acting that made me more confident and also a lot happier. You are going to learn those same techniques as you work your way through this book. Those techniques allowed me to become the person I was meant to be. We are not meant to be insecure and self-conscious, hiding ourselves away and not believing in who we are or what we have to offer. The spiritual teacher Marianne Williamson wrote that 'Your playing small does not serve the world. We are all meant to shine as children do. As we let our own light shine we give others permission to do the same.'

Babies, puppies and kittens all have such enthusiasm for life. They don't shy away, they like being the focus of attention, they expect us to like them and we do. True inner confidence is really all about liking yourself and feeling good about who you are, not having to try to be someone else or to big yourself up and not needing to impress others or work to make them like you. But confidence is not arrogance; they are so different because arrogance is the opposite extreme of lacking confidence. Arrogant people are just trying to convince themselves and you that they are someone, but if they really believed it they would not be concerned with or care about what you thought of them.

Confidence can be a quiet self-assurance that radiates from you. It's like when someone knows that they are good with children or animals, or a natural cook, dancer, athlete or painter: they don't tell you how good they are, they just get on with it. Children and animals can't be fooled: they know if you like them, if you can handle them, and it can't be faked. You can learn to have a genuine and authentic confidence about the things you are naturally good at. We are all put on the planet with a talent. Everyone is good at something, but it's important to remember that you are not meant to be good at everything. People who know they have a talent don't try to be good at anything else; they know it's enough to be good at one thing and they feel confident about how good they are, too.

Years ago my partner had prostate cancer and he had been to see one particular specialist who said, 'Well, I will do my best; we have to see how you respond to treatment, we must hope it works but there are no guarantees.' I persuaded him to see another specialist who was considered to be the best prostate cancer specialist in England. He ran some tests and then said, 'I can help you, you will survive this, you are in the best hands. I am the BEST prostate specialist in Europe.' I can't tell you how good it was to hear that; it was reassuring rather than arrogant and his confidence made me feel so much better and helped my partner to make a full recovery.

Similarly, when I was on a flight once that hit really scary turbulence the pilot came over the airways and said, 'I'm sorry that I am giving you an unexpected Disney ride here but, don't worry, I am a very experienced pilot, one of Delta's best, and I know how to deal with this. We will be through it soon.' Again, his confidence was welcome and made us all feel better. We didn't think the pilot was arrogant or conceited; we were reassured by his confidence. People don't dislike confidence and confident people – they love it. If you rang up Gordon Ramsay and said, 'Gordon, I am coming for dinner at your restaurant tonight; how do I know the food will be good?' Gordon would probably reply, 'I am the best f***ing chef in the world; it won't just be good it will be bloody marvellous.' Most people, including his staff, really like and respect him. He doesn't say he's also very good at gardening or painting, he just states that he is good at one thing: food. It's his passion, and it's great to have a passion for something.

I used to take my daughter with me to give food parcels to homeless people, which was a great thing for her and me as when we came home we were so grateful for everything we had. Just having a house, a bed and a fire made us feel like royalty and so lucky. The organisation I belonged to that helped the homeless would try to get them off the streets by offering them work. When they asked them what they were good at they would run off a long list: I am good at carpentry, gardening, I am a chef, I am a builder, plumber, janitor, driver, mechanic, handyman etc, etc. What they were all saying was 'I am a jack of all trades and master of none'. But really you only need to be good at one thing and what you are naturally good at lies behind and is connected to what you love to do, so find out what you love to do and be amazing at it.

Jane Asher began her career as an actress and then used her creativity to become excellent at designing and making cakes and writing many successful books showing us how it's done. She is an excellent example of someone who only needs to be good at one thing: she is a fantastic baker who only needs to focus on cakes. It's her niche and she does it brilliantly. Kim Wilde and Monty Don both switched careers and made a success out of their passion for gardening. People who love what they do would do it for no salary if they didn't need one. When you do what you love your confidence soars; on the other hand, it's almost impossible to feel good about yourself when doing things you hate.

In Step 5 we will focus on what you love to do and what your natural gifts are, but please don't skip ahead to that part as this book is written in a very special format that changes your mindset chapter by chapter, so read it in the sequence in which it is written to get the best and most permanent results.

Confidence-affecting Triggers

One of the rules of the mind is that feelings will ALWAYS overcome logic as they are so much more powerful, so it stands to reason we have to change the feelings rather than the logic. We have to change the feelings that make you hold back and fear taking risks or taking action. This is exactly what you are going to learn to do. By changing the feelings about putting yourself forward, being the centre of attention or speaking to strangers, those actions will cease to be a worry to you and you will find you can enjoy them. You can be as at ease with attention as a small baby is. You won't have to work to make it feel natural; it will feel and be natural. It is so empowering to be happy in your own skin.

You may think it's odd to refer to a baby's or a child's confidence, but children are constant reminders of the innate confidence we are born with. When my daughter was four and I used to drive her and her friends to school, I would often say, 'Who can sing?' and they would all put up their hands and say, 'Me, me, I can sing, I am really good at singing' and then sing songs for me, and it was so sweet to listen to them singing out of tune and getting all the words wrong while believing they sounded perfect. If I had asked them to sing when they were fourteen they would all have shifted in their seats in discomfort, rolled their eyes in mock horror and ignored me while my daughter would have told me off for being embarrassing and childish and showing her up in front of her friends.

By fourteen they have acquired a fear of being judged – and of being judged badly – that simply does not exist in infants. No one can judge you except you yourself and as you learn to judge yourself really well you will succeed in acquiring and keeping Ultimate Confidence.

My five-year-old niece is a natural athlete and will proudly tell me, 'No one at school can catch me. I am the fastest runner.' She is also incredible at tennis and has already been marked out as a gifted player and she spends all her free time hitting a racquet; it would not occur to her to play her ability down. When I said to her recently, 'I hear you were the best in your school', she said, 'No, I was the best out of six schools.' She said it without arrogance, just as a statement of truth. She hasn't been told don't brag, don't show off, don't be big-headed, and she has not experienced the envy or resentment of siblings or classmates that can make a talented person feel uncomfortable.

But as we grow up this changes and we start to adapt to people's responses to the way we present ourselves to others. When my daughter was eight she came second in her school at sports day and was given a badge stating this. When I said to her, 'That's so fantastic, you came second out of the whole school', she immediately began to play it down, saying, 'Well, Mummy, some of the children in my school are only five so it doesn't really count', and I said to her, 'Don't do that, don't lessen what you have achieved. You came second out of the whole school and that's amazing and I am proud of you.' She was already learning to play down her achievements.

Feeling good about your particular talents, skills or interests is exciting and liberating. You experienced this once. You may not remember, but you did. You came into the world wired to succeed and loving an audience. You said the word bicky and your parents responded with 'You said the word biscuit, you are so smart, here's your biscuit, you clever thing.' You pointed to a ball and said the word ball and everyone ran to get it for you. You got clapped and praised for walking, talking, pointing and smiling. You even got a round of applause for peeing in the toilet, and when you got things wrong and mispronounced words, or got food in your hair, or put your shoes on the wrong feet, or forgot to put your pants on when you dressed, your parents thought it was so cute they even took pictures of you like that. And then siblings came along or you went to school and the praise did not come so quickly; you really had to earn it and other kids could do things you couldn't do better and faster than you. Your failings got pointed out and no one thought it was cute, or sweet, or endearing any more. When I took my daughter into her classroom one day she pointed out another five-year-old and said, 'She can write her name neatly inside a box and I can't.' I replied, 'Well, sweetie, her name is Mia and yours is Phaedra and that's much harder to write neatly than Mia. When you're older no one will care or even remember who could write their name first, everyone will be able to do it. But you are so good at drawing and not everyone can do that.' It bothered me that her first school measured the children's progress against each other even at five and only rewarded results, not effort, which is damaging for small children's self-esteem.

I spent my teens and twenties feeling like a failure although I actually had fantastic successes and I was offered so many opportunities that I turned down in case I was not good enough or failed. It was only when I began to study hypnotherapy while living in Los Angeles that I discovered how easy it was to regain real inner confidence. Through the ground-breaking discoveries I made during more than twenty years of working with clients as a therapist on television, radio and in my own clinic here and in America, I devised a simple and effective way to show people that they can be confident, they can really like themselves and they can have personal success. You will find my methods very different you will also find that they work.

It is an unfortunate truth that to underachieve you have to have a belief system and convictions about yourself which hold you back from the person you are meant to be; these beliefs must be uncovered and erased for good. We are all programmed to act and react in certain ways; human behaviour is not random, it's quite predictable. You are simply going to reprogramme your attitude to yourself so that it is the one you were born with, not the one you have acquired through poor role models and incorrect beliefs and advice.

BREAKING NEGATIVE BELIEFS AND HABITS

It is very important to question all of your negative beliefs. Why do you believe you are not good enough? Where does that belief come from? Who first told you that and what did they know anyway? What did they base that inaccurate assumption on? Some of the most successful people were told they would never succeed. Elvis Presley was fired from the Grand Ole Opry after his first performance and told to return to truck driving as he didn't have what it took and would never be a singer. The Beatles were turned down by Decca; J. K. Rowling's first book, *Harry Potter and the Philosopher's Stone*, was rejected several times; Albert Einstein was diagnosed with a learning disability and labelled incapable of being educated. Thomas Edison, who became the greatest inventor of our age, was expelled from school and labelled not smart or worthy of further education.

Some of the most successful and wealthiest people today were diagnosed as not very bright or capable. Gordon Ramsay was let go by Glasgow Rangers Football Club due to injury. Simon Cowell and Peter Jones (of *Dragons' Den*) both started at the bottom, worked their way up, lost everything then started again and now enjoy huge success and wealth. Felix Dennis went to prison after publishing *Oz* with two colleagues; he got a shorter sentence because the judge considered him 'very much less intelligent and therefore less responsible' than the other two co-defendants. After his release he became a publishing tycoon and multimillionaire, worth an estimated £750 million today. He was allegedly so offended by the judge's comments that it drove him to prove himself.

Our beliefs change all the time. When you question a belief you start to doubt it and no longer hold it to be true, but you need to make sure your beliefs change for the better. When working with clients who lack confidence I look at their beliefs. The same beliefs come up over and over again:

- I have always been insecure and self-conscious.
- I have never been confident.
- I have been shy all my life.
- Everyone in my family is self-conscious like me.
- I have tried but I just can't pass exams.
- I am no good at interviews.
- I can't talk to someone if I like them or am intimidated by them.
- My relationships never work; I only seem to attract losers.

These beliefs cannot actually be true, but if you continue to talk about yourself like this then you are continuing to be a part of the problem instead of being part of the solution. Even if they were true you can change a belief which in turn can change your confidence, because your beliefs affect the physical processes in your body. In other words, every thought we think creates a physical reaction in our bodies. Our thoughts affect our blood flow, which is why we can blush at a mere thought. Thoughts can create anxiety and tension, increased blood pressure and heart rate and your thoughts can and do have a powerful effect on your self-esteem. The process is as follows:

- Your thoughts control your feelings.
- Your feelings control your actions.
- Your actions control your behaviour.

So, you see, your thoughts affect and control everything but they are *your* thoughts and you are free to change them easily and instantly. This book will show you how. Channelled properly, motivational thought processes can be more powerful than pharmaceutical drugs. I am going to show you how to change the images, words and beliefs you run in your head on a daily basis and this in turn is going to permanently boost your confidence and increase your self-esteem.

Exercise 1

The Magnet Test
If you want proof of how your thoughts run your body, here is a fun test.

Stand up with your feet slightly apart and your arms by your sides, close your eyes and begin to imagine that just behind you is a huge magnet pulling you and rocking you backwards. Really focus on the magnet; see it as a huge U shape with the red paint on the ends just behind your shoulder blades. Say to yourself the magnet is pulling me backwards and you will feel yourself swaying and rocking and tipping backwards. Now imagine the magnet has moved to just under your chin pulling you forwards; again, as you think about the magnet pulling you forwards, your own power of thought will cause you to rock forward, to sway forwards. Now imagine the magnet has moved to the left of your left shoulder and find your body is being pulled to the left; then, as you imagine it to the right of your right shoulder, notice your body swaying in that direction, and, of course, the more you focus on the magnet, the stronger the pull will become and you can just notice that happening.

If you prefer you can close your eyes and ask a friend to describe a magnet behind you, then in front of you, then at either side of your shoulder or ask someone to read this section to you.

Of course there is no magnet in the exercise above, but you are beginning to see and to feel for yourself your mind's ability to accept whatever you tell it, whether real or imagined. As your mind accepts the thought of the magnet it goes to work to have you react to the magnet, even though it only exists in your imagination.

The same is true with every thought that you have. If you think of failing your mind makes a picture of what that looks like and then works to make the picture a reality. Fortunately, it does the same thing when you think of succeeding. If you think of being forgetful or of having a fantastic memory the same thing happens, so one thought can generate positive reactions and another thought will generate negative reactions within the body. Whether these thoughts are based on fact or fiction is irrelevant to the mind because it cannot tell the difference.

Exercise 2

The Weight Test
Here is another safe and simple exercise to prove to you that thought really is the most powerful thing. You can do this sitting or standing. Close your eyes, stretch both hands out in front of you at shoulder height and close both hands as if

you are holding something in each hand. Now begin to imagine that in your left hand you are holding an enormous red fire bucket filled with about fifty pounds of heavy, wet sand; feel the weight of that bucket in your fingers, feel the weight moving up to your wrist, your elbow and now your shoulder, feel it getting heavier and heavier by the second and notice that your arm is being pulled down by the weight of the bucket. The more you focus on the bucket, on its heaviness, its colour and size and contents, the heavier your arm is becoming and the more it is being drawn downwards.

As your left arm continues moving downwards, imagine that you are holding in your right arm the hugest helium-filled balloon, see the balloon's bright blue colour, see it as almost bigger than you are, feel the string in your hand and, because helium is lighter than air and because this balloon is firmly held in your right hand, you will notice that your right arm is moving upwards, lifting upwards, travelling up higher and higher, becoming lighter and lighter, almost floating upwards of its own accord. As you think about the balloon and bucket notice the difference in your arms: one is heavy, one is light, one is moving up, the other is moving down and the cause of this is your thought process.

You may prefer to memorise this or to have someone read this part to you, as you keep your eyes shut. Again, the point is to show you how easy it is to influence your mind, and to prove to you that thoughts have a very real effect on our bodies.

Thoughts effect chemical changes in the body. Positive thinking can produce chemicals in the brain and cells of the central nervous system, which then affects the immune system. This can then produce NK (natural killer) cells, T cells and white blood cells, which can destroy certain types of illness and fight bacteria and viruses and keep us healthy and resilient.

Because the strongest force in the mind is its need to make us act in ways that match our thinking it is vital to change any negative thoughts and beliefs about you and your capabilities.

So you must focus on how you want to be, never on how you don't want to be. In other words, keep your mind on what you want and off what you don't want.

Focus only on what you want to move towards and accomplish, never on the opposite, which is what you want to leave behind.

This becomes easier as you find the flip side of every negative thought and use that instead.

- Whatever we focus on we move towards.
- Whatever we focus on we experience and feel.
- Whatever we focus on we get more of; it becomes more real to us.

If you focus on having an injection and watch as the needle goes in you will increase the pain sensation, but if you focus on something else, like reading something engrossing, you may not even notice the sensation of the injection. If you focus on fear it increases, like when we watch scary films late at night, but if you focus on deep breathing you become calmer.

Another rule of the mind is that we are what we think and believe. For example, if you're reading this book but are already convinced that it won't work and that programmes like this don't work for you then you must turn these negative thought patterns around. You have not been on this programme before because it is unique and cutting edge and it absolutely will work for you. Permanently.

The Different Types of Confidence

Throughout this book you are going to find solutions for every type of confidence issue and for all the feelings that go along with not liking yourself as much as you could including:

- LACK OF CONFIDENCE
- LOW SELF-ESTEEM
- POOR SELF-IMAGE
- ATTRACTING THE WRONG RELATIONSHIPS
- NOT GETTING PROMOTION
- POOR SELF-WORTH
- INSECURITY
- PROCRASTINATION

There are different types of confidence lackers and each type uses extreme behaviour, activity and energy to mask insecurity.

The types fall into three main categories but the cure is the same for all of them: they need to like and accept themselves as they are, to take the risk that when they can just be themselves they will be at peace and then their self-esteem will increase.

Type One – Holding Back. People who hold back include those that are Shy, Insecure, Nervous, Procrastinator, Quiet, Studious, Own Worst Critic. They are better at relationships than careers and use hiding away to mask a lack of confidence.

Type Two – Pushing Forward. People who push themselves to the front include Arrogant, Aggressive, Bully, Diminisher, Bragger, Superior, Extreme Optimist (the I-am-always-right-and-never-wrong type). They are better at careers than relationships. They use aggressive behaviour to mask an extreme lack of confidence.

Type Three – Acting/Hiding behind a Mask. People who create a mask to hide their true selves include Grandiose, Comedian, Workaholic, Perfectionist, Control Freak, Extrovert, Vain, Wacky Dresser or Immaculate, Perfect Dresser.

Whatever category you may put yourself in as you work through the exercises in this book, old feelings of self-doubt and insecurity will be banished as you increase your sense of self-worth, self-value and self-image. In turn, everyone around you will also increase their sense of your worth, value and image. Your mind remembers the feeling of achieving and being happy with yourself and you can reactivate and re-create that through this programme. Since you were born wired to succeed and to achieve and to like yourself you will find it easy to relearn habits that already exist within you and once you have reactivated them you can keep them forever.

How to Change

The first stage in changing our attitude and our confidence levels is to be aware that nothing in life *ever* influences human beings more than what they link pain and pleasure to, and then using this information to our benefit. Changing what you link pain and pleasure to and choosing what to link pain and pleasure to can and will change your whole life. Moving towards pleasure and away from pain is a survival instinct. This means that every single time you experience pleasure your subconscious mind searches very fast to find the cause of it, your brain then stores the cause of that pleasure and reminds you of it next time it becomes aware you need to feel pleasure. When you experience pain (any pain, physical or emotional) your mind searches even harder for the cause of the pain. It locks on to and remembers that cause (even if you don't) and then does everything it can to stop you moving towards that pain again. Your brain is programmed to constantly move you towards pleasure and away from pain and it will always do more to avoid pain than it will to find pleasure; avoiding pain is how we survive on the planet so the subconscious mind is highly motivated when it comes to avoiding pain.

Since our greatest need is to be accepted and our greatest fear is to be rejected, many of us avoid pain by avoiding situations where we could be rejected, such as not talking to someone we are attracted to in case they don't feel the same. Or not asking someone for help in case they say no and not going for a job we really want in case we don't get it. One of the most important lessons I ever learnt was to stop fearing rejection. Learning that and putting it into practice was such a gift to me; if I had not learnt that

I wouldn't be writing this book now as I would be too scared that my editor would not like it and would give it a terrible review or, even worse, the publisher would laugh at my efforts and it would never get published.

The only risk in life is to not take the risk; not taking risks is the biggest gamble of all. I have met people who told me they wrote a book but did not submit it in case no one liked it, or had an idea but did nothing with it for fear of rejection, only to watch as someone else took a similar idea and became successful with it. Others tell me they really felt an attraction for someone but didn't ask them out in case they rejected them, only to watch as that person ended up with someone even less confident than them.

Many years ago I worked with someone who wanted to be an actor and when I asked him what he was doing about becoming an actor he said, 'What should I be doing?' and I replied, 'Well, at the very least getting an agent, going to acting classes and going to auditions.' He then said, 'I can't do any of that. I can't walk into an audition because I am too scared of being rejected and I am too nervous.' I knew then that it was unlikely he would make it as an actor unless he could overcome his fear first. Acting is a business in which there is huge rejection and the only way actors cope is to not make it personal – the best actors don't read bad reviews. I bought one of my actor clients a cushion embroidered with the words 'There has never been a statue erected to a great critic' after he had been mauled in the press, and it made him feel better.

If you write, paint, design, perform, give a presentation or do anything that requires an audience you will find some people love it, some don't, some will reject your work, others won't, but they are not rejecting you, so you don't need to link pain to it and thus avoid doing what you want to do. Some people even get anxious about buying a gift in case they get it wrong and the other person doesn't like it and thus doesn't like their taste. Many people can't return food in a restaurant or an item in a shop or ask for their food to be prepared differently in case the waiter or shop assistant doesn't like them. **By changing what you link pain and pleasure to, and by seeing that no one can reject you, you will stop avoiding situations and live a fuller life.** As well as becoming more conscious of what we each link pain or pleasure to, we also have to consider the confused messages we give ourselves by linking both pain and pleasure to the same thing, since this causes huge problems for our mind, too. Our brain becomes confused because it can't move us towards pleasure and away from pain when they are linked to the same thing simultaneously. Your brain is like a missile moving you away from pain and towards pleasure. When you link pain and pleasure to the same item it becomes like a tumble dryer going round and round and getting nowhere, and this confusion will affect your behaviour.

I have many conversations with my clients who have not pursued their goals because, instead of linking pleasure to succeeding and to going out and making it happen, they link pain to all the potential rejections and nos they might come up against. When you link pleasure to getting a pay rise or a promotion but pain to having to ask your boss for it, you will be stuck. You link pleasure to having a fantastic career but pain to the interview process or the long hours you would have to put in, and pain to the fact that you would have to get up early every day and pain to missing out on your free time or your social life.

If you link pleasure to being in a loving relationship but could not go into a bar alone, or talk to a stranger, or put your details on a dating site in case someone laughs at you, you are also stuck. If you link pleasure to eating chocolate and pain to going on a diet you will stay overweight. Even when you have a great relationship the pain of being rejected does not end; sometimes it can increase. If you really love someone and they leave you, the pain of having to go through that again in a new relationship can be too much for some people who make a decision that they would rather be alone than be dumped or rejected ever again. Loving someone and being parted from them can also cause enormous pain.

When you think like this your brain is busy doing everything to make sure you avoid pain and your brain is going to win, but since it's your brain this programme is going to make sure you use it in a way that makes you win at having lasting and liberating confidence.

You cannot succeed at anything if you simultaneously link pain and pleasure to it. If there is anything in life you really want and don't have, it's because you link more pain than pleasure to having it. When I work with patients who have problems conceiving it is often because they link pain to being pregnant, pain to the birth and pain to the disruption a new baby can cause, and while they still desperately want a baby their mind's job is to move them away from what they link pain to – being pregnant and having a baby. One of my clients who had problems conceiving due to control issues and then got pregnant decided that she would give birth at home while her husband banged a drum, burnt incense and they chanted together. She was very proud of her birth plan and told me it was going to be magical and natural and she would squat and give birth easily, like a Native American. She linked pleasure to the idea of a drug-free home birth and pain to the idea of a hospital birth. When I saw her some weeks later I asked her how it went and she said, 'Oh, my God, it was so painful. Why didn't anyone tell me? I abandoned the home birth and made my husband drive me to hospital and begged him to get the doctor to make me numb from the neck down. When he said, "But what about your birth plan and our natural birth" I screamed at him, "F*** my birth plan, this f***ing hurts. Get me anaesthetised now."' She immediately reversed what she linked pain and pleasure to and we can all do that just as instantly. An example of a similar situation in your life would be if you hate hospitals or taking painkillers, and avoid all medicine, and then find yourself in pain. If the pain is bad enough you will take any medicine. You will link pleasure to getting the medicine instead of pain; you will go to hospital to get pain relief and you may even thank the doctor for scheduling you. You will have reversed what you link pain and pleasure to. Reversing it is easy and I will show you how to do it and how to make it last a lifetime.

Only humans can choose what to link pain and pleasure to. It is their major advantage but it can also become their major disadvantage. A cat cannot choose to link pleasure to having a bubble bath any more than a polar bear could choose to link pleasure to being on a beach in tropical heat, and a lion can't choose to link pleasure to becoming a vegetarian. You can choose what to link pain and pleasure to and in doing so you can succeed or fail to have the life and the confidence you want. You have enormous power to choose what to link pain to. Now that you realise just how effective this power can be, use it consciously and to your advantage to link pain to living an unfulfilled life and to avoiding situations that you might actually end up enjoying. At the same time link a huge amount of pleasure to achieving all your goals, having high self-esteem, liking yourself and being happy.

Everything we want in life, with few exceptions, is because of how we think it will make us feel; you need to make yourself feel good about going for your goals instead of fearing how you would feel if it didn't work out. **You cannot fail; you can only fail to try.**

Once you remove the fear of failing you have stopped linking pain to it.

You can reverse what you link pain and pleasure to and you can make it permanent by following the exercise opposite. Using the sentences opposite as a guide, write out what you link pain to and then change it or minimise it so you cannot link as much pain to it ever again, which in turn will stop the confusion in your mind and stop you procrastinating and putting things off. By minimising or changing what you link pain to and maximising what you link pleasure to, you are already reversing your pain and pleasure cues and you are already beginning to change your life for the better.

Exercise 3

Write out what you link pain to, for example:
I might not succeed.
I could fail.
I might look stupid.
I could be rejected.
If I don't make it I won't be able to cope.
People might laugh at me.
My work might not be good enough.
I might find out I have no talent.

Turn that into pleasure:
I will succeed, I will make myself succeed, this programme is wiring me to succeed.
I can't fail, I can only learn more about me and get another step closer to my goals and finding out what I am meant to do.
No one has the power to make me look stupid.
No one can reject me unless I allow them to and I won't do that.
I can cope with anything as I move towards my goals.
I am more than good enough.
Everything that doesn't work out takes me closer to my real talent and abilities.

Now write out what you link pleasure to, for example:
I will get my promotion.
I feel great about asking for a pay rise and do it with confidence.
I am comfortable talking to strangers; people like me.
I am ready to attract the right person into my life as I feel good about myself.
I am excited about discovering my talents, gifts and abilities.

There are many studies from schools where children were told they were gifted or extremely talented and became outstanding students because of these beliefs. The pioneer of this was an amazing American teacher called Marva Collins who has had studies dedicated to her and papers written about her ability to get the most disadvantaged children to believe in themselves. She even had a film – *The Marva Collins Story* (1981) – made about her extraordinary ability to motivate impoverished children to get way above average results, and she also received the National Humanities Medal for her particularly inspiring teaching ability. She said, 'Success doesn't come to you, you go to it' and '**There is a brilliant child locked inside every student**'. Her studies between students with similar academic levels found that the ones who liked themselves always got better grades.

Similar studies from hospitals show that patients who believed they were given a special healing medicine or drug would make remarkable progress. Placebo drugs were based on these studies.

When a military training academy tested results based on the belief system of trainee cadets they found that trainees who dropped out had pessimistic beliefs and would blame bad luck, or bad tuition, or fate as a reason for failing whereas the positive cadets put their success down to their personal approach to life, their high self-belief and positive attitude.

STEP 2

'*No-one can make you feel inferior without your consent*' –
Eleanor Roosevelt, US First Lady

Your Greatest Needs

- We need to be accepted, but first you have to accept yourself.
- We need to not be rejected, but no one can reject you unless you let them.

We all have a fear of rejection and a need for acceptance; however, no one can reject you without your permission or consent.

Humans all have the same needs; worldwide our greatest need is to be accepted and our greatest fear is to be rejected. Sometimes when I explain this to clients they respond with 'Oh, I don't fear being rejected. My greatest fear is losing my money or my job', and I point out that when you lose all your money or your job, position and status you feel rejected.

Your fear of being different and not fitting in and belonging makes you the same as everyone else as we all feel different to some degree and we all fear not belonging. We have this fear because we are tribal people and our survival is linked to being accepted and belonging to the tribe or the group, which in turn meets our need to feel safe and secure. If the tribe rejects, banishes or casts out a member he or she may not survive.

In the television series *Tribe*, Bruce Parry joined tribal communities in remote places around the world to experience their way of living. He always behaved just like the tribe: he dressed (or went naked) like them, ate the same food as them even when he hated it, and very quickly got them to accept him as just like them. When people see us as the same rather than different they like us and accept us; if we feel different they see us as different and don't accept us. Animals do this too – they like you if you feel at ease around them and will become anxious if they pick up your unease, which makes them dislike you. Since we no longer live in tribes our survival is no longer linked to being accepted in this way, which means that no one can ever make you feel rejected unless you allow them to. When you fully accept and like yourself you will find that other people accept you too.

When you increase you own sense of self-worth and self-image everyone around you will increase their value and perception of you as well, plus it's much harder for anyone to reject you when you do this. We must belong; our survival on the planet is linked to belonging but we already belong just by being here. The key is not to try to belong or try to fit in but to feel comfortable enough in ourselves to feel good about being around other people and to radiate that out to others. This book will show you how to do this so you are a walking, talking affirmation of what you believe, which is that you belong, you fit in, people like you and you like yourself.

If you fear rejection and need acceptance you are just like everyone else on the planet, but the truth is no one can reject you unless you agree with them. In order for someone to reject you they have to believe something about you which is going on in their mind, not yours. You have to believe everything they believe in order to allow them to reject you.

One of my favourite stories is of a journalist going to inter-view a holy man; the journalist rubbished all the beliefs of the holy man and insulted everything the holy man stood for. Throughout the insults and criticisms the holy man continued to smile, even to beam, with happiness and contentment. Finally the journalist said in exasperation, 'I don't understand why you are smiling. I have just criticised you and mocked you.' The holy man replied, 'If you offer me a gift and I don't accept it, who has the gift?' 'Why, I do,' said the journalist. 'Exactly,' replied the holy man, 'I don't accept your criticisms. They belong to you and they can stay with you.' You can apply this to being criticised: if you don't let it in and if you don't accept it then you leave it with the critic.

I told this story to one of my clients who had a particularly horrendous family. During a subsequent appointment he told me that his mother was furious that he was no longer dependent on her for approval, and on his last visit had said to him, 'I hope you die of cancer.' He calmly replied, 'Oh, Mum, that is so mean. I am not even going to let it in.' I was so proud that he got it: that she could not affect him with her criticisms unless he was in agreement with her. So if people try to diminish you and put you down, see it as an item they are trying to give you that you won't accept and is therefore left with them. **Not letting in criticisms and insults is one of the most beneficial things you can do to boost your self-esteem.** Learning to say, 'I am not going to let that in' or 'I am choosing not to let that in' will help you to grow in confidence. You don't need to return or trade insults if you don't accept them in the first place.

I have worked with so many people whose greatest problem is that they feel different from other people, that they don't feel the same as others. It's exactly the way I used to feel. Feeling different can be the bane of our lives. It's self-perpetuating. We have to think it and believe it and then it resonates out from us to others who radiate it back to us. Sometimes when I am working with teenagers who are telling me how awful they feel, how no one understands them because they are different, I ask them to poll all their friends and to ask them if they also feel different or not the same. They always come back astounded that almost all their friends feel the way they feel, so if you feel different from everyone else that feeling means you are the same as everyone else.

When I began to work on television I knew the deal: some people like you, some don't. Having worked with so many celebrities I was well aware that being in the media is not all about being accepted and approved of; it's also about being rejected and criticised. When I first appeared on *Celebrity Fit Club* one redtop newspaper wrote that someone should send me a razor to shave of my moustache. I was a little bothered when I read it but I know that I don't have a 'tache and, if I did, believe me, I would be having it bleached or waxed off right now. I realised it was the lighting on set that made my upper lip look darker and decided to forget about it . A year later that very same paper wrote a very complimentary review of me and my book. They could not have been nicer.

When I appeared on *Celebrity Fit Club USA* I got some particularly vicious hate mail from other women saying things like, 'Your legs are too thin, you must have had liposuction. You should not be on the show because you are a fake.' I decided to imagine the life of the person who wrote that letter to me and the effort they put in to trying to make me feel bad about myself, and I was glad I wasn't them. I figured that whatever they think I look like they must look even worse and I felt okay about it.

If someone said to me, 'I don't like you or can't get on with you because you are a punk rocker or a goth and I hate them', I would just assume they were slightly nuts and ignore them. It's no different from saying, 'I can't get on with you because you are a Martian or a Hell's Angel, heavy metal fan or you have green hair and I hate that.' You would not allow such bizarre comments to affect you so therefore you have the power to not let any comments in, including being called a bitch, tight-fisted, boring, stupid, ugly, fat, dead wood, useless, hopeless, a waste of space etc. **The mind can and does refuse to let in what we choose not to believe, so by choosing not to believe those things your mind simply won't let them in.**

Change Your Thoughts to Change Your Confidence

If you truly believe that people like you they will, because another rule of the mind is that the universe will support everything you believe. However, if your belief is that you don't fit in you will constantly look for proof to back up your belief and you will find it. If you believe people warm to you and get to like you as they get to know you – or, even better, if you choose to believe that people like you straightaway because you are so easy to be around and such good company, so relaxed and assured – then you will look for proof of that and, again, you will find it. Obviously you do have to really believe it – it won't work if you just try to believe it or try to make others believe it.

One of the universal rules is that we find proof of our beliefs everywhere we go. This has been scientifically proven with people who believe they are lucky and experience more luck statistically than those who feel unlucky. People who like themselves get stopped more often in the street by people asking the time or for directions? That's because they have a more approachable demeanour and they look confident and therefore appear more likely to know. Studies showed that testers asked random strangers for directions and one in twenty of the testers touched the stranger on the arm or hand at the end as they thanked them. When the strangers were polled they remembered almost everything about the stranger who touched them and they liked them. We like people who make contact with us as long as it is appropriate and does not invade our space. People need to be connected to other people and being touched by others and touching someone is a powerful way to do it. No matter whether the touch is a warm handshake, a congratulatory pat on the back or a genuine hug, people respond to touch. A recent experiment looked at waitresses and waiters to see if touching customers influenced the tips they earned.

The first group of waitresses/waiters touched each customer on the arm as they took their order or as they delivered their food. The second group of waitresses acted in a warm and friendly way but they did not touch the customers. What the researchers found later was that the waiting staff who touched their customers earned 50 per cent higher tips than waitresses who did not. The customers perceived the touching waitresses as more likable, confident and open; they liked them because they liked themselves and thought different and better thoughts about themselves.

The human brain produces approximately 50,000 thoughts a day. Sadly, most of us think the same thoughts today that we thought yesterday and will think the same thoughts again tomorrow. Changing your thoughts can and will change your life. I have met so many people with what I call misdirected confidence: they are certain they can't do something and convinced they will never be good at anything and will always fail. They have a powerful belief that they will fail or be rejected and because the belief is fixed it tends to be realised. This is a kind of confidence: it's just confidence that you will fail and needs to be turned to confidence that you will succeed. You can see that whatever you believe becomes true; if you believe you can't do something you are right, and if you believe you can you are also right. We make our beliefs and then we go out into the world looking for examples to back them up and we find them. Whatever you choose to believe you will always find an example to support your belief. You can experiment with this by deciding to believe for one day that people are dishonest or mean and look for examples of that everywhere you go; the next day look for examples of how honest or kind people are. In each experiment you will find proof of your belief. When you change your beliefs the universe will support your changes and prove you right. **Remember: first you make your beliefs and then your beliefs make you,** so make sure your beliefs are good ones that will help you, not hurt you, that will motivate you and propel you forwards rather than hold you back.

Why Rejection Can Be the Best Thing to Happen to You

When it all changes. We come into the world certain that all our needs will be met, since they were in the womb, where we had everything on tap. We also come into the world unaware of what rejection is and then it can all change. I have often found, working with patients, that so much damage is done when an authority figure has diminished them as a child, put them down, criticised them and made them feel worthless. Sometimes it's a parent, relative or step-parent; sometimes it's a teacher or an older sibling. My father was a teacher and you could not find a kinder and more understanding teacher on the planet. However, some teachers really should not teach and some of them teach because they have been thwarted in their chosen career. I worked with a champion gymnast whose coach disliked her and constantly diminished her because she had so much more talent than him. I worked with a stunning woman who never had relationships because her headmaster humiliated her in front of the whole school. She had been caught with another child looking at each other's genitals and, instead of the headmaster recognising that small children often do this, he shamed them both by making them stand in front of the whole school, stripped to their underwear, while he castigated them for being depraved and dirty. I also worked with a brilliant CEO who did not understand why she always felt so bad about herself, until we traced it back to every school report saying 'useless, talentless, will never amount to anything'; and with an actor who could never remember his lines and had an issue with authority figures because he was caned in front of the school for something so trivial. At his school boys were not allowed to have their hands in their pockets and he kept forgetting this. As a result his headmaster decided he must be touching himself so he caned him during assembly while telling the school he was depraved and disgusting.

Apparently the actress Kate Beckinsale said that she was never allowed even to be in the drama class at school as her teacher told her she had no talent or acting ability. The singer Sophie Ellis Bextor was also told she had no singing talent. Luckily neither individual paid any attention to the criticism. Greta Scacchi's teacher told her to take her head out of the clouds when she discussed her desire to act. When I was at school my PE teacher told me I was hopeless at PE and had absolutely no coordination or ability. She would not let me be in any of the school sports teams so when I appeared on *Newsnight* demonstrating aerobics, and became one of the most successful aerobics teachers in London, it pleased me to imagine her watching it. I loved it when Will Young sang The Doors' song 'Light My Fire' on *Pop Idol* and Simon Cowell told him it was 'distinctly average'. Will immediately responded with 'Simon, I don't think you could ever call that average.' He didn't say it with arrogance or with any sense of being deluded about his talent. He didn't argue or get aggressive; he simply stated what he knew. He had delivered an impressive rendition of 'Light My Fire' and would not allow Simon to diminish it. Simon then reconsidered and agreed with him. So, you see, even Simon Cowell can be swayed by someone who won't let himself be rejected. Paul McKenna often mentions that his teachers told him he would amount to nothing. How wrong they were.

When we are young we are incredibly vulnerable to such damage, but as adults we have options when it comes to the way we deal with rejection, including rejection that occurred in the past. Catherine Zeta-Jones was apparently devastated when a relationship ended so she moved to America, partly to recover from it, and there she met and married Michael Douglas and became Hollywood royalty. She must be so grateful that she was rejected since she would not be where she is today without that rejection. Piers Morgan was fired from the *Daily Mirror* under a cloud, yet he is more successful than ever. When Robbie Williams was fired by Take That he was written off; again, he went on to even greater success. When Gordon Ramsay was let go by Rangers he went on to enjoy far greater success without them because he became free to excel as a chef. These are rejections that they might be thankful for.

I used to have a fabulous job at one of London's most prestigious dance studios but while I was abroad on holiday a misunderstanding occurred and I lost my prime-time slot, which was pretty devastating as I loved my job. Unwilling to start at the bottom again, I went to another dance studio sure that they would employ me as I was known as one of the very best teachers. However, they turned me down, so, feeling even more rejected, I went to a third, much less prestigious gym and they offered me a job on the spot as their best teacher had just left to train Princess Diana. Within weeks of taking that job I had met the love of my life in that new gym and within six months I had moved to Chicago with him. If I had not been fired then rejected (twice) I would not have met him or moved to America and my life would not have changed as fantastically as it did.

When I was in my teens I was rejected and dumped by a boy who caused me much pain. Years later he contacted me and asked me to meet him again. When I met up with him it only took a few hours before I said in my head, 'Thank you, God, I am so, so grateful he dumped me or I would still be with him and this would be my life and I am so grateful that it isn't.' When my second book got rejected I went on to get a deal that was many times better than the first one that had been withdrawn. When I was trying to buy my first flat I was gazumped and when I found my dream home and the deal fell through I was bitterly disappointed. However, I found another house that I didn't like nearly as much and that I did not really want, but since I had already exchanged and would be homeless I had to move, so I bought it, remodelled it and it turned out to be better in every way than my dream house. I used to drive past the dream house and think, 'Wow, am I glad it didn't work out.' I love my house; it's so much nicer and better than the one I lost out on.

I can look back at some major rejections in my life and see that, although they hurt me at the time, in the context of my life they were good, even great, for me and I would not be where I am today without them. If your first boyfriend/girlfriend had not dumped you, if your first boss had not fired you, where would you be now? It's worth you doing this. Take a few moments and imagine that the first person who dumped you hadn't and you are still together, you didn't get fired from that first job and you are still in it.

In the TV series *The Apprentice*, Ruth 'The Badger' did better by being rejected than hired as she went on to get her own TV show, *Badger or Bust*. By not working for Sir Alan Sugar she was free to take up press and media opportunities that the winner, Michelle Dewberry, could not. I think Claire Young, who came second on the 2008 show, will go on to do much better than the winner. She has already gone to work for Karren Brady at Birmingham City Football Club.

On many other reality shows the person who is rejected often achieves greater success. For example, Liberty X did so much better than Hearsay on the show *Popstars*. Darius Danesh was voted off *Popstars* and was voted out of the top 10 for *Pop Idol* then got reinstated when Rick Waller fell ill and ultimately came third, and long term did better than Gareth Gates, who was placed second. Lemar has achieved so much more success than both winners of *Fame Academy*. G4, who lost out on winning *The X Factor* in 2004, went on to have more success than the winner that year. Duffy, who is now a huge star, was rejected on the Welsh *X Factor*.

The *Big Brother* contestants who have had lasting success are not always the winners. Alison Hammond, who was voted out first on *BB4*, has gone on to great success. The Twins and Chantelle have already done better than the winner of *BB8*.

Have you ever had to reject someone, i.e. had to tell a guy or a girl that you did not want to see them any more and that they weren't right for you? Did you enjoy every minute of it or was it awful, and you were glad when it was all over? Very few people enjoy rejecting someone. When I was dating and it wasn't working I absolutely hated having to tell someone that I didn't want to see him again, that he just wasn't right for me. I have also been on the other side, when I was told I wasn't right and the person didn't want to see me any more, and I don't think they particularly enjoyed it either. I have also been fired and been in the position of having to fire someone and, again, I hated firing people and I didn't find the people who fired me having a great time while they did it.

Having to reject someone is painful and being rejected is painful, much more so if you take it personally. If you have ever forgotten to return a call you know that you were not sitting at home gleefully rejecting someone; you simply forgot to call them. And when someone forgets to call you, remember how easily it is done and decide to know that they are NOT busy deliberately rejecting you; they just forgot.

Although reality TV shows would have you believe that we love firing people and celebrating their discomfort, very few people genuinely enjoy this.

Moving On and Letting Go

In order to be happy and at peace with yourself you must be able to:

- Forgive the past.
- Feel great about the present.
- Feel really excited and positive about the future.

It's so important to move on from any painful events in your past in order to lose the negative influences and effects they have on you. To move on you have to be able to forgive the past, feel grateful for the present and feel excited about the future. Being grateful and forgiving are essential steps on your journey to liking who you are. The future is perfect, innocent and unsullied but we are capable of carrying into the future all the unresolved pain of the past and tainting our future. It's what I call the luggage of life; some people carry around so many old resentments and hurts that they don't need and it pollutes their future unnecessarily.

Letting go of the past and forgiving solves this. The significance of any event is linked to how well and how honestly you can deal with it and mourn any loss that occurred. If an event such as a death, a hurt or a rejection is not dealt with and the feelings about that event are not expressed the event will linger on in our consciousness and cause us a lot of pain.

Here is how to express yourself: forgive, let go, move on, have high self-esteem and BE HAPPY.

The most important words in the world are Let Go. You cannot move forward while holding on to old resentments and hurts, so forgive people not for their sake but for yours, so that you can move on.

If you have been diminished here is how to get over it for good:

Exercise 1

Imagine the teacher/relative/critic is in front of you. I want you to tell them how you feel and, before you decide this is silly and skip it, it is <u>essential</u> that you do this because those feelings are either kept inside you or out of you and you will be better and do better when they are out of you. One of the reasons doctors ask mothers to write a letter to a stillborn baby is because they recognise how much damage unexpressed grief, hurt and anger can do. '**The feeling that cannot find its expression in tears, may cause other organs to weep**' is an expression from way back and is as true as ever today.

In American courts the practice of having the victim or victim's family give an impact statement to the judge and perpetrator was found to be so incredibly healing that it was extended to allowing victims to meet their attackers in jail and tell them how they felt. By being allowed to express their feelings of anger, hurt and pain they were able to be heard, to get closure, to let go and to move on. This also worked when a Japanese prisoner of war met his torturer and forgave him: he wrote a book about it, *The Railway*

Man by Eric Lomax. It also worked when an IRA terrorist met the daughter of the man he killed. Simon Weston met and befriended the Argentinean pilot who bombed him during the Falklands War.

This exercise really works so don't dismiss it. Do it and discover the benefits for yourself. All my clients tell me that doing this was especially beneficial and allowed them to move on and finally get over the anger, the hurt, the resentment and the effects of being put down or treated badly.

Start by saying Mr/Mrs/X/Mum/Dad etc.
I need to tell you that I deeply resent how you treated me.
You had no right to do what you did.
You were absolutely wrong to behave that way.
I did not deserve that.
Add anything you like.
Tell them how much better you are than them.
Tell them what a great kid you were.
Say you must be such a sad person to be so mean and I am sorry for you.
Add some swear words, very important because small children can never say you were a f****** prat to an authority figure. However, saying it as an adult makes you feel so empowered as you are doing something a helpless child could not do, saying something a defenceless child could not say.
Ask them how their life has turned out and remind them that since you would not want to be them even for a minute you have already won.
Tell them that you would never do that to a child so you are already a better person.
Really think about this as you do it. Give it your all because you will get so much back, including being free from holding on to resentments.

The Common Denominator of All Problems

As a therapist I noticed very quickly that the common source and cause of a lack of confidence is believing you are not lovable and not good enough. All children come on to the planet certain they are lovable and with a confidence that their needs will be met. We are all born with a belief that we are lovable and good enough just as we are, and that belief is not lost but submerged beneath newer beliefs that we are not good enough, pretty enough, smart enough, successful enough, rich enough etc, that we are not lovable just as we are.

I have met plenty of gorgeous, talented, wealthy, even hugely famous clients, who felt utterly unlovable. It did not matter how much other people believed in them, they had no belief in themselves so they felt worthless. I frequently meet people in my practice who want to be confident but believe they have never been confident and feel that confidence is something that eluded them from birth. The truth is all babies are born with innate self-confidence and with high self-esteem. If you bring a newborn home, put it in a cot and shut the door. It will cry for hours until someone comes to attend to it because babies have a belief that says, 'Someone will come and attend to all my needs because I am worth it.'

When I used to take my baby out in her push chair, strangers would come up and coo over her, reach into the pram and tickle her chin or feet, and I was fascinated by the fact that she never looked away or found all the attention too much. She was never self-conscious or remotely fazed by being the centre of attention, she lapped it up, smiling and laughing; her behaviour said, 'I like this attention and I am worth it.' When you hold a small baby in your arms and feed it, it will stare at you for ages and not break your gaze. Babies don't look away and get uncomfortable with all the attention; they soak it up. Babies look at people with complete ease because they have not acquired a reasoning that says, 'Why is this person looking at me? What's wrong with me? I don't like being looked at.'

Last year on holiday I was listening to the children around the pool saying, 'Daddy, watch me jump in the water, Mummy look at me swimming, Mummy, Daddy, Granny look at me, look at what I am doing.' They were all saying, 'Pay attention to me because I am worth your attention.' We were all like that once and it's a shame we have forgotten how to fully believe in ourselves and our abilities. Many adults feel very uncomfortable being the focus of attention. They don't like being looked at for long periods of time and have no idea that they came into the world loving attention and believing they were worth it and certain that they were lovable. Through this book and audio download I am going to activate the same beliefs you were born with – an absolute knowledge and feeling of certainty that you matter, that you are lovable and confident. And while you're subconscious mind recreates those feelings and beliefs your conscious mind will let go of all the acquired negative feelings that you don't need.

When you're born you only come through your parents not from them. The universe created you. The universe is your family and the same universe that created you will support you in everything that you do, especially in knowing that you are lovable. Even if your parents did not appear to want you or value you, there are people in your life who want you to be here and you are here for a reason with something valuable to offer. I work with so many people who desperately want a child and would be loving parents, and yet for some of them it never happens and is tragic. I also work with people who have had horrific parents who did not deserve the children they had. It's not easy to make sense of that except to accept that we are meant to be here and our parents are the people we come through but not from. Someone wanted us to be here, something wanted us to come on to the planet as ourselves.

I read a story about a man who, aged thirty-two, bankrupt, jobless and having just endured the death of his young daughter, decided to kill himself. But as he stood on the shore of Lake Michigan summoning up the courage to drown himself, he heard a clear, distinctive voice in his head say, 'You do not have the right to eliminate yourself. You belong to the universe. Your significance may remain forever obscure to you, but you may assume you are fulfilling your role if you apply yourself to converting your experiences to the highest advantages of others.' He was so shocked and moved by the words that he wrote them down and began to do as the voice told him. That man was R. Buckminster Fuller, who went on to huge riches and phenomenal successes financially, professionally and in his personal life. He invented the geodesic dome (now used at the Eden Project and the Epcot Center) and he also helped countless people. I love that story because it re-enforced my belief that we all belong and that we are all here for a purpose.

Nature never re-creates anyone. There is no one else in the world exactly like you, hasn't been before, isn't now and never will be again anyone on the planet quite like you, and that means that you are here for a purpose with something to offer. When you find out what that something is you will feel so much better about yourself. As you work through this book and do all the exercises, you will find out what that something is and you will be happier, more at peace and become your healed self instead of your hurt or damaged self.

It's important that you recognise yourself as unique instead of special. People who feel special feel alone and isolated. You are unique but also just like everyone else on the planet so you can feel connected and feel the sense of belonging that we all need.

When you are little you need Mummy and Daddy to love you; in fact, your survival is linked to your parents loving you – if they have an attachment to you they will nurture you. In turn, children idealise their parents, often way beyond the level that nature requires of them in order to survive. But our unquestioning belief in them at a young age can also cause pain and hurt, because we believe our parents are always right even when they appear not to love us. We are left assuming there is something wrong with us not them. The reason for this is that we are dependent on our parents; if we work out that they are inadequate we can't cope with that realisation because it threatens our safety and survival. Instead, it's safer or easier to believe that we are at fault. As a result we try to change to make it better, but of course that doesn't work because we are not at fault. This inability to change things, to make our parents love us, leads us to feeling helpless and hopeless; unable to change anything and even more certain that we are unlovable. These feeling begin in childhood but may persist into adulthood, tainting our future. It's time to clear that up once and for all. You are not and never have been unlovable. Parents do the best they can even when that is not enough or woefully inadequate; no parent wakes up thinking, today is the day I am going to ruin my child's life, and then sets about doing just that.

As a child the most important words you hear come from Mummy or Daddy or a teacher. As a grown-up the most important words you will ever hear are the words you say to yourself and believe, and the most important opinion is your opinion. As a grown-up you don't need your parents love or approval; you might want it but you absolutely don't *need* it. The following exercise will help you realise that.

Exercise 2

To really implement this I want you to imagine that you go to the home you were raised in, walk down the path, go in the front door and up to your bedroom. In that room is you as a little child. Pick up that child and take them back to your home where you live now. Take them on a tour of your home and show them all the things you have that you did not have then, all the things you have accomplished and the freedom to do what you want. Show them all the clothes in your wardrobe that you choose, the products in your bathroom that you use, the food in your kitchen that you buy, your CDs and DVDs, your books and magazines –

---

everything that is in your home now that was not in your previous home.

I want you to repeat some things out loud to that little child. Don't worry that they sound a little cheesy; just do them because it works.

While you imagine holding the very young you in your arms, I want you to say:

I am becoming a loving parent to you now.

No one in the world can play this role like I can.

I love you exactly the way you are and I always will.

I am here giving you all the love, praise and recognition that you are entitled to.

You are safe with me I am here protecting you and loving you always.

You are a part of me and can never be rejected or abandoned because I am a part of you and you are a part of me.

I will never ever leave you; you are safe, valued and loved always.

Make sure you have installed the younger you in your adult world, then I want you to write out all the things you most wanted to hear when you were little and then say them to yourself many times a day until they sink in and stick. Remembering those words, think of all the things you really wanted to hear, most needed to hear and would have loved to have heard, and say them to yourself right now and continue to say them to yourself on a regular basis until you fully feel the benefits. Say the words you were entitled to hear. It's not difficult; we pretty much all want to hear the same thing, words like:

You are a great kid I am so lucky to have you.

You are so lovable.

I love you just the way you are.
I am so glad you are my son/daughter.
You are so pretty/smart/wonderful/intelligent/lovable/cute.
You are so wanted.

Add whatever works for you. Don't just think it or say it and move on; really do it and then stick your words on your mirror, or screen saver, or in your wallet so you can keep reading them and start believing them. We are all a walking, talking affirmation of what we believe about ourselves so changing what you believe about you is a vital step on your journey to lasting self-esteem. I used to be amazed at the amount of successful, accomplished grown men who would cry during hypnosis when I said some of the above statements to them. Just saying you are a good son or a good person would make them weep because they had never heard those words and so needed to hear them. Don't wait any longer. Fill yourself up with those words, do it now and keep repeating them. We all talk to ourselves all the time so you are only doing what you already do but in a more productive and effective way.

The exercises you have just done are designed to free you from needing parental love or approval and to stop you in any way, either consciously or unconsciously, from feeling emotionally stuck and to instil in you all the good feelings you may have missed out on in your childhood. Many of us at an emotional level are stuck in our childhood and by moving the child into your adult world and showing him/her that it's a good, safe and better place you are moving on unencumbered by the past. The following exercise is to prove to you that you no longer need your parents to love you in order for you to be happy.

Exercise 3

Imagine your parents have moved in with you to make amends and spend every moment telling you how much they love you, how proud they are of you, praising you, doing special things for you, making you your favourite meals, hugging you and making up for all the stuff they did not do when you needed it. They just want to be around you, spending all their free time with you, telling you how much they love you, love you, love you and admire you. How long would it take before you were longing for them to move out? A few days, two weeks tops.

If you really do this and fully use your imagination you will find that you have just proved that you don't need your parents' praise, recognition and love any more and now you can move on and give yourself all the praise and recognition that they were unable to give you. I have done this exercise with clients thousands of times and over twenty years I only found one client who said, actually, she would like her parents to move in with her for good and it would make her happy. She had not seen them since she was three so I understood. But you and I understand that it would not and could not make an adult man or woman happy to live with their parents for ever. Most people say, 'Oh no, I would hate that. I love my parents but that thought is horrible.'

It's ironic that so many adults are affected by the fact that their parents did not love them enough, yet as an adult if you were still living with loving parents in your forties it would actually mean that you had failed to succeed at creating your own life. No one at forty wants to take holidays with their parents or go out for the evening with their parents, and, while it is lovely to take your parents on a trip or outing, if they were your constant and only companions you would be showing the world that you had failed to move on and make other successful relationships

Everything Is Available to You

When I was working on a chat show in America a woman called in to talk to me. She was very distressed and in order to relax her I asked her to imagine walking on the beach with the sand between her toes. She replied, 'I have never been to the beach. I live in the middle of America and the beach is not available to people like me. It's way too far away and I can't afford to get there.'

I have never forgotten her reply: 'It's Not Available To People Like Me.' It had a profound impact on me and as I work with clients I notice how often they believe that being happy, having someone to love them, being successful, having money, even having peace is not available to them. Just because it was not available to you as a child it does not mean it is not available to you now. As a child, having a car, your own credit card, your own home and holidays of your choice, even choosing what to do at the weekends, were also not available to you but that does not mean these things are not available to you now. If you think like that you must give up that belief immediately. Here's how.

Exercise 4

I often ask my patients to think of all the things that are available to them now that they did not have as a child. You can do that right now. As a child you can't choose what to eat, what to wear, what time to come in, even when to go to bed, but as an adult all those things and so much more are fully available to you. Think of all the things that are available to you now that were not available in your childhood

---

like foreign travel, having your own money to spend, driving a car, wearing whatever you like, having a mobile phone, DVDs and CDs, magazines, a digital camera, jewellery. Even basic things like having the choice of what TV channel to watch, when to eat, what to wear, what time to go to bed and get up. As you recognise just how much is available to you as an adult that simply was not available to you as a child, you can now think of all the other things that you are not accepting as available to you.

The benefit of doing this is that, as your mind understands just how much is available to you as an adult that was not available as a child, it will shatter the belief that says:

It was not available to me then.

It's not available to me now.

It will never be available to me ever.

When I worked with overweight people who were not allowed sweets or chocolate as children they still continued to believe that they were not allowed them years later. They would go to the shop and buy sweets and eat them very quickly, not really enjoying them or tasting them, and they would feel really guilty and think, 'I should not have eaten those, that was bad, I am bad for eating them', which would perpetuate the binge eating even more. They would eat so-called naughty or forbidden food quickly and guiltily, just as they had done as children, even if they lived alone and no one could see them, because of the predominant belief that it was not available to them and therefore they could not or should not have it. Even though they may have eaten chocolate as adults every day, the belief that it was not really available to them was more powerful and damaging than the behaviour of eating it. Making these people see that chocolate would always be available to them and they could have it whenever they wanted to, but that they did not need to, was enough to end the behaviour.

People who rarely receive praise can become so unaccustomed

to it that if you say, 'You look lovely' they will respond with 'What, in this old thing?' or 'I can't look nice. My hair is dirty and I have spots.' If you say to them, 'You did a great job' they will reply, 'Oh, it was nothing really. Anyone could have done it.' Some people are so unaccustomed to being praised that they feel acutely uncomfortable with praise and have to reject it and replace it with a criticism. Not allowing someone to pay you a compliment is like not allowing someone to give you a gift. If someone gives you a compliment accept it and say thank you. That way you are letting it in.

When we rarely get praised and often get criticised we seem to continue the behaviour, rejecting praise and criticising ourselves. Like all learned behaviours you can stop this at any time by deciding, 'Okay, I did not get praised as a child. Does that mean praise is not available to me now or ever? No, of course not.' By praising yourself on a regular basis and remembering when you were praised by others you are breaking that belief.

The saddest thing is people who believe that love is not available to them because it was not available to them as children. Marilyn Monroe was rejected by both her parents and went through life believing that real love was not available to her, yet the public loved Marilyn. Even so, she could never fully accept that love was available to her. She once said, 'I knew I belonged to the public and to the world, not because I was talented or even beautiful, but because I have never belonged to anything or anyone else.'

We are all programmed to re-create and seek what is familiar to us and we seem to feel most secure and comfortable with what we know even if it's not good or right for us. That's because our subconscious mind is programmed to recognise and attract what is familiar rather than what is desirable. To move on, make the familiar unfamiliar by changing your thinking. Just because you may be familiar with rejection or criticism, or not having money or enough love, that does not mean you have to continue it. We don't continue to eat baby food just because chewing was once unfamiliar; we get used to anything over time. Our parents or grandparents did not have indoor toilets or central heating but we are totally used to them. Most teenagers today cannot imagine life without a mobile phone. Before I had a car it was absolutely normal for me to take the bus everywhere and I did not find it a hardship, but once I had a car I got used to it and found buses less attractive and definitely less enjoyable than going door to door in the comfort of my own car. Think of all the things you once did not have and now do have and you will realise how quickly you have adapted to things that were once unfamiliar and unavailable to you. Every time you go on a summer holiday you adapt to heat. The fact that you are not used to living in a hot climate all year round does not mean you can't adapt to it. Human beings can get used to anything as long as it is consistent, so you can get used to consistently believing in your confidence and worth by using the methods and techniques in this programme.

STEP 3

'You may be disappointed if you fail, but you are doomed if you don't try' – Beverly Sills, 1929, US opera singer and fundraiser

You Don't Have to Be Perfect to Be Confident

You are not meant to be perfect; perfect people simply don't exist and those people who try to be perfect are the unhappiest people in the world. They have entered a race to be perfect that has no ending, and as they get close to the finishing line it continually moves further away from them. Trying to be perfect or trying to make your life perfect is an illusion as it is not possible, but the quest for it will cause you much unhappiness and stress. If you believe you will be confident and happy when you look, act or feel perfect, or when your partner or children are perfect, or you are perfect at your job, you are setting yourself up for major disappointment and unhappiness. I am often asked why some of my clients, like supermodels or top movie stars, would need therapy when surely they have it all. Being beautiful or talented does not protect people from suffering. They are in a competition to stay beautiful and it's a competition they have to enter every day of every year. One of my clients who got an award for being the best actor said it put him under tremendous pressure to get the same award next year. Being on the best dressed, best looking, most talented lists brings on the pressure to stay there. Patti Boyd said that when she saw herself on the cover of *Vogue* she could only see every flaw and fault. Many of my clients who became very overweight were unconsciously opting out of the competition to look good as it was too stressful and it's a full-time job with no days off.

People who are beautiful know it doesn't last but it is their identity and they are lost without it, which is why so many iconic beauties become reclusive as they age; Marlene Dietrich, Ava Gardner, Rita Hayworth, Greta Garbo and Brigitte Bardot all chose to spend their older years out of the public eye. Elizabeth Taylor allegedly said people came to see how old and fat she had become and she never disappointed them. Brigitte Bardot said she gave her beauty and the best of herself to men but she gave the rest of herself to animals as they never judged her.

My friend who is a television executive told me the five stages of celebrity are:

Who is Rita Hayworth?

Get me Rita Hayworth.

Get me a younger version of Rita Hayworth.

Get me a Rita Hayworth type.

Who is Rita Hayworth?

In my twenty-four years as a therapist I have noticed that the happiest people are those who aim to be the best they can be but also accept that they are real, flawed people having relationships with other real, flawed people. Nothing is better than knowing someone loves the real you; when they love the perfect you they are always going to be disappointed. When someone loves you because you are beautiful, what happens when your beauty fades? There is a famous story about Laurence Olivier giving the most amazing performance as Hamlet that had the audience weeping. He received a record number of standing ovations and when he left the stage the press rushed to his dressing room to interview him. He met them looking stone-faced and told them not to write about his performance. When they asked him why on earth not he replied, 'I don't know where that came from and if you write about it and everyone comes to see it they will only be disappointed if I can't be as good as that again.'

Many of today's anxieties and stresses come from feeling we are not good enough and have to do more; whether it's improving our appearance or what we achieve, we live under constant pressure to be and do more. Performance anxiety is a name for the anxious state people put themselves into before they go for an interview or take an exam, or even for the kind of situations that put us on the spot in everyday life – some people become deeply stressed if they have to talk to a stranger or make a particular request for something, and some children or young people can develop performance anxiety at school or college.

The anxiety comes from the feeling that we are not interesting enough, or funny enough, or smart or attractive enough. You don't need to be funny – after all, some of the funniest comics are hard work and a mass of insecurities when they are offstage. I have worked with many comedians who are often quite hostile, bitter and cranky because they feel they have to be funny and perform all the time. It's amazing how many comedians suffer from depression – Tony Hancock and Kenneth Williams killed themselves – and how many of their wives say they are never funny at home and can be hard to live with. Always having to be the wit, the raconteur or beautiful or fascinating means you can never be yourself or be loved for who you really are.

Some of the most intelligent people are not natural communicators – many geniuses find it hard to communicate, and deeply intellectual people can find it hard to fit in. What makes us like a person is not how smart or funny someone is but if they are warm and genuine and whether we can relate to them or they can relate to us. I know I have already said this but I am repeating it because the mind learns by repetition: 'We like people who are like us, who we feel an affinity with.' When I was sixteen I used to baby-sit for a five-year-old girl who was a genius. One night as I put her to bed I asked her to call me if her baby brother cried and I didn't hear him. She replied, 'Well, I won't call you in case you don't hear me either. Instead I will flash it in Morse code on the garage door and you can see it through the window.' When I told her I did not understand Morse code she looked at me with such pity and said, 'Really, how old are you?' 'Sixteen,' I replied. 'Well, I shall proceed to teach you,' she volunteered, but very quickly gave up. She was so much smarter than me but I didn't envy her. Another time I was reading her and her brother *The Tale of Peter Rabbit* and she constantly stopped me to say, 'Rabbits can't really talk, they don't have vocal cords, you know. Rabbits don't wear coats, they have their own thermostat and they don't have the coordination to put on clothes.' She was an enchanting little girl but very isolated as other children could not play with her. She was too different and they could not relate to her. When I was pregnant with my daughter I didn't wish for her to be a genius. I wished for her to have a sunny disposition as I knew it would give her a good life and lots of friends. If you stop and think about why you like your friends you will find that it's because you can relate to them and you feel comfortable with them. The basis of all friendships is that *'we choose people who share our vulnerabilities'*, we pick people who are like us; your friends like you for the very reason that you like them and you never have to try to impress people who already like you.

When we are first making friends at infant school, and later when we are dating, we all go thought the ritual of my favourite food is, my favourite colour is, and we love it when our friends agree. Later we move on to my favourite novel is, my favourite film is, my favourite band is, because that's how we connect to people and it's how they connect to us.

How to Deal with Critics

Critical people always have the most criticism reserved for themselves but express their own dissatisfactions with themselves outwardly by finding fault and criticising others. When I was newly engaged my female boss said to me, 'Your boyfriend is so gorgeous. How do you keep him?' I was shocked by her comments but I replied, 'I keep him the same way he keeps me.' Years later another person said to me, 'Your boyfriend is so unattractive. What are you doing with him?' Rather than arguing or being annoyed, I replied, 'Isn't it great that he's got so much going for him that he's really attractive to me? He's an amazing person and that's why I love him.' In each example the critical person obviously had some need to make me feel bad because she felt insecure or unhappy and in both those situations I chose not to let it affect me because I knew it was not really about me.

As well as this issue that leads people to criticise is the fact that in general we feel the need to feel equal to those around us in order to belong, and, as I said before, our survival on the planet and our security are linked to belonging. So imagine the metaphor of being on a seesaw with someone and you are higher than them and they are lower than you. For the person who is lower than you and wants to be equal to you, the easiest thing they can do to restore the balance is to embellish themselves or diminish you to change the dynamics of the seesaw. They may want you to be lower on the metaphorical seesaw, in which case they will try to diminish you and put you down or embellish themselves until they feel better than you.

I find the most effective way to deal with them is to say to them or think to yourself, 'This is not really about me it's about you', or 'You must feel really bad about yourself to be like this', or I just say to myself or to them, 'You know, when you keep criticising other people you are just showing me and them how dissatisfied you are with yourself.' It is not always appropriate to say these things to your boss or relatives but nothing can stop you thinking them and there are times when it's okay to say them, but always say them in a calm, rational, non-confrontational way.

People who like themselves like other people; people who don't like themselves don't like others. It's not possible to like anyone more than you like yourself. The definition of high self-esteem is how much you like yourself. You simply cannot have one without the other.

Believing you are lovable is not arrogant. You are finding acceptance of yourself which is a powerful means to gaining lasting confidence, whereas arrogance involves trying to convince others of something and thereby showing up a lack of self-belief. Remember, when it comes to arrogant people, the person they are trying to convince the most is themselves. Arrogant, bullying or aggressive people are extremely insecure deep inside themselves and put on a show to hide and to fool themselves as much as to fool others. Bullies are usually very insecure and unhappy inside but hide it with aggressive, domineering behaviour. One of my clients was bullied at school by another girl who was very mean to her. In order to help her cope I got her to practise saying to the bully, 'You must be really unhappy to be like this' and 'You don't like yourself very much, do you? I feel sad for you.' She said it every time the bully targeted her and, to her surprise, one day the bully capitulated and admitted that she was really unhappy. Her mother had cancer and her home life was a mess. The bully decided my client was the one person who understood her and decided to become her friend. It was not what we had in mind but it was interesting how the dynamics of that relationship changed when the bully felt understood and could get a friend in a way that did not involve intimidation. I often work with young children who are bullied and always recommend saying to the bully, 'Oh, you don't like yourself today', 'You're unhappy.' I know these expressions sound glib but they work because bullies don't like themselves, they are always unhappy and they can't be themselves because they feel no one would like them if they knew the real person.

If you have to deal with a bully *never, ever* do anything that says 'please like me'. Your behaviour always needs to say, 'I like myself and I don't need you to like me.' When we act in a way that says, 'I need you to like me, please like me, what can I do to make you like me?' the balance of the relationship is always in the hands of the other person. If you are dating someone it's also very important to look at what your behaviour says; it's great to do nice things for the other person because you like them and they like you, but again you must avoid behaviour that says 'please like me', 'I am working hard to make you like me.' We like people who like themselves and if you have to work extra hard to make someone like you that says you don't like yourself enough. Your behaviour needs to say 'I like myself' rather than 'I need you to like me'. Working to make someone like you is *not* the same as working to make a relationship and friendship last by putting in time and effort to be together and doing things for each other. Often when I work with patients who seem to veer from one bad relationship to another I get them to ask themselves just one question. 'How do I feel about myself when I am with this person?'

If the answer is 'I feel less than' or 'He/she is better than me, smarter than me, much more attractive than me, too good for me, I feel inferior to them' or the worst of all 'I just don't feel good enough for them', then it's time to do some work on yourself and end that feeling or find someone who does not make you feel that way.

If the bully is your boss you can still find strategies to deal with them. It really helps to understand that at work being respected is more important than being liked, and in relationships being respected is as important as being loved. I worked with someone once who was spectacularly rude to me and then justified his behaviour by saying, 'I don't like you' and I replied, 'I don't need you to like me, I already have great friends, I only need you to respect me.' He then said, 'I talk to everyone this way' and I said, 'That's up to them but I don't let people talk to me like that.' Eventually he stopped being quite so rude because I didn't allow him to undermine me or make me feel bad about myself. We all show people how to treat us all the time and it gets easier to make others treat us with the respect we deserve if we can calmly stand up to them.

I also had an issue with someone pressuring me to tell them

something confidential that I did not feel comfortable telling them. When I initially said I didn't feel comfortable discussing it, they replied, 'Well, I can talk you through the discomfort' and what really worked was to say, 'I am sorry but I can't make your need to hear this, more important than my need not to tell you.'

Some people who like you the way you are will be unhappy about the changes you will experience from following this programme, especially if they lack confidence and are envious of your new-found confidence. We like people who are like us and people who feel inadequate feel comfortable with people who also feel inadequate as it's reassuring to share the sentiments. Your friends or partner or family may resist you changing as they may feel threatened, or feel that your confidence highlights their lack of confidence. But once they see what you have gained, and how easily you did so, they may be inspired by your changes and feel your positive impact on themselves.

How to Silence Your Inner Critic

No matter what the previous critics in your life were like, the most destructive critic in your life today is **you**. You are much harsher on yourself than your boss, your ex or any old adversaries. The way we talk to ourselves, the words we use and the tone of voice have a powerful effect on our emotional state and it can make us or break us. You need to use your own voice to build yourself up not pull yourself down. There are enough critical people in the world and you don't need to be one of them.

Superior people give praise to others, while inferior people criticise. Criticism withers people whereas praise builds them up. If you leave the house without your keys or map or directions do you say, 'I can't believe how stupid or dumb I am, I'm an idiot' or are you nice to yourself? Do you say, 'Oh well, I made a mistake. I won't ever do that again and I can still find my way there.'

If you make a big mistake it's unlikely you will repeat it as you learnt something. I only ever locked my keys in my car once as it cost me so much to call out the AA that I learnt to be careful from then on, and I conditioned myself to make checks to ensure it couldn't happen again. Similarly, when I stepped outside my front door late at night to put out the rubbish wearing only a T-shirt, and the door shut behind me, it caused me so much embarrassment that I have never repeated that mistake. Your critical voice is supposed to help you by saying things like 'Don't forget to, don't go there, don't do that, remember to____'. It's not supposed to say, 'You idiot, have you got shit for brains, you dumb loser, stupid moron' or words to that effect.

The most important words you will ever hear are the words you say to yourself and believe, so stop putting yourself down, because you are human and make mistakes. Instead, realise that the only way we advance and improve in life is by making mistakes and learning from them. The most effective way to learn anything is by making mistakes. That's how we all learn. If you don't make a mistake you won't learn, so don't feel bad or beat yourself up about the mistake but instead remind yourself that you are learning in the same way everyone else does. Napoleon said, 'A man who never made a mistake never made anything.' When I was living in LA I was learning Spanish and did not understand that the word 'take' in the context I was using it meant take as in sexually taken, so when I told my boyfriend's mother in Spanish that I would take her shopping in my car I actually said to her in front of everyone 'I will f*** you in my car'. I said it several times as she looked so confused and I thought she did not understand my Spanish. Only when someone else pointed out my mistake did I get why they all looked so shocked. I have never made that mistake again!

Part of liking yourself is respecting yourself and the way to do that is to silence the inner critic and to use praise instead of contempt for your actions. An example would be:

- I forget to return that call and it was really important. I am so hopeless. I can't get anything right. What's wrong with me?

Change it to:

- Thank goodness I have remembered it now. I can still return the call and they will understand.

- I meant to put credit on my phone/pay my bill. I have a terrible memory, my mind is like a sieve and that's going to cost me late payment charges. I am such a dum-dum.

Change it to:

- Okay, this doesn't work for me so I am going to set up a direct debit so that can't happen again.

- I forgot to charge my phone again I am a moron and I never learn.

Change it to:

- I am going to buy a car charger/keep a spare charger at work/in my briefcase so that will never happen again.

One of the reasons babies and toddlers have high self-esteem and natural confidence is that they don't have a critical voice that says:

- I spilt my food, I am an idiot.
- I peed my pants, I am an embarrassment.
- I just can't do it. I can't get the hang of walking. I'm a failure.
- I just can't get it right. I am hopeless, useless, stupid.

Babies believe that they are lovable in spite of their behaviour. If you do the same you will feel the same, so imagine you have never had a critical voice and end the self-criticism. To stop the critical voice you don't have to DO anything, you have to STOP doing something that has been proved to be harmful, hurtful and damaging to your self-esteem and confidence; so turn off, shut down and end your inner criticism and you will be a different person and you will have better relationships with those around you too.

Imagine if you lived with a friend or partner who made a point every day of telling you what your faults were and what you were doing wrong. How do you think you would feel if they stood over you while you were cooking and said, 'That's wrong. You've ruined it now', or commented as you got dressed, 'You look awful. You look a complete mess', or as you worked at your job said, 'You just blew it. You can't get anything right'. We all know what it's like to drive with a passenger who says, 'You have gone the wrong way, you should never have taken this route, you are going to be late now, you need to overtake, you are going too slow, you will never fit in that parking space.' Wouldn't you want to kick them out of the car or maybe just kick them out of your life? The thing is, you are doing that to yourself every day and you need to stop it. If that was your friend you would get a better friend, so be a better friend to yourself and build yourself up instead of putting yourself down. From now on any time you say something negative immediately stop and just change it to something positive. By being positive about yourself you will grow in inner and outer confidence.

When my daughter was about fourteen it became a common thing that she would leave the house for school only to return five minutes later, and I would always say, 'What have you remembered?' instead of 'What have you forgotten?' It was good that she remembered so quickly and came back to get it within five minutes, and I didn't want her to come back feeling she was forgetful and a failure. By saying, 'What have you remembered?' I was telling her she had a good memory not a bad one.

Every time you say, 'I have a hopeless memory, I haven't got a clue. My mind has gone blank; my mind is like a sieve' you are making a statement, and since the strongest force in all of us is that we turn into our expectations, whether they are good or bad you are literally contributing to making your memory worse. If you say, 'It will come to me any second now, I will remember it because I have a great memory' then it will.

We have all had that experience where you say to yourself, 'What is the name of that great restaurant I went to, that film I last saw?' When you ask yourself such questions your mind goes straight to work, finds the answer and pops it into your head. Your mind is set up to come up with an answer to every question you ask it.

Ask it, 'What was the name of that book I read last summer?' and it will find the answer.

Ask it, 'Why am I such a loser? Why am I a failure? Why can't I get anything right?' and it will answer those too.

Ask it, 'Why does it always go wrong?' and you are telling your mind to justify why that statement is true. Your unconscious mind will find answers to those questions. Your unconscious mind is designed to simply answer questions, which is why questions such as 'Why do I always mess everything up?' will cause your mind to search for and find an answer to why you always mess things up.

When you say, 'Why am I a failure?' your mind will answer with something equally negative. That sentence is a statement: 'I am a failure. Why?' It's not a question. To grow in confidence and self-esteem ask your mind specific and positive questions and you will get specific and positive answers. By simply replacing 'Why?' with 'What can I do to?' 'How can I find a way to?' you are programming your brilliant brain to find an answer to it.

An example is if you say to yourself, 'Why am I alone?' Your mind will answer, 'Because no one likes you.' Turn the negative into a positive by asking your mind, 'How can I find my soul mate?' and it will give you a specific answer in the form of solutions, such as do voluntary work in an area that interests you so you can meet like-minded people.

When you say, 'Why am I fat?' your mind will answer the

question with 'You eat too much.' Ask it, 'How can I become slimmer?' and it may come up with something like stop eating wheat because it knows you are intolerant to it.

Ask it why you never succeed at interviews and it will answer with because you are not good enough. Ask it, 'How can I come across really well in interviews?' and it will respond by coming up with solutions like 'Who do I know who does come across well and could they advise me?', or it might tell you to get some coaching.

This probably sounds almost too simplistic but your mind is like a computer. It comes up with the right answers when you give it the right questions. The more specific you are the better the answers. So for your next exercise change any negative statements to positive ones and instead of making negative statements ask specific questions.

Example:
- Why am I always broke?
Change it to:
- How can I get a job that pays more?
- What do I need to do to increase my earning potential?

- Why am I such a loser?
Change it to:
- How can I increase my confidence and self-esteem?
- What are my natural talents and abilities?
- What am I really good at?

If you want to be confident ask confident questions, and if you want a better life ask better questions. Changing **why** questions to **how** questions will have an amazing effect on your life. It's another simple change that has huge and positive effects on your life.

Another very effective way is to listen to criticisms from yourself and others and then talk back to them by adding *according to whom?* or *thanks for sharing your opinion/viewpoint even though I don't feel the same way*. You don't need to argue with critics; just don't let the criticism in. When you are the critic you can ask yourself 'Where does this opinion come from?' Who taught it to me? What did they know? Do I have to believe it?' The answer is NO. You have a brilliant brain and you have a choice. You can use it to rationalise why you feel so bad or you can use it to talk yourself out of it. Always do the latter and you cannot fail to become more confident.

If it's your own critical voice it's very useful to turn it into the voice of Mickey Mouse, Tweety Pie, Eeyore or Wallace & Gromit and laugh at it. By making the voice comical it loses all its power. You can also imagine that the critical voice is like a radio in your head and you can turn the volume down to silent. It is also useful to just say to the inner voice, 'Shut the f*** up!' At times this is highly effective.

When I was on holiday a little boy came out of the pool and his grandma immediately began to say, 'You have not dried yourself properly, you will get a cold, you should not have gone in the pool so quickly after lunch, you might get cramp, you should not talk to those people they are strangers.' He was obviously completely used to this because he just looked at her and said, 'Grandma, Back Off.' He was about six and had already found a way to deflect her criticisms. My friends and I laughed about it but I thought it was a great comment. You can say things like that to yourself: back off, cut it out, go away, be nice, be kind. It is not just what you do that builds self-esteem; it is also what you don't do or cease doing. Stop criticising yourself and you will build up your confidence and your self-esteem. When you stop criticising yourself your self-esteem is raised and you become aware that it is not your performance or your behaviour that makes you feel bad but the critical way YOU speak to yourself about it on a regular basis.

A well-known therapist told me a very amusing story of a client who was impotent. When he asked him what he heard in his head as he got undressed prior to sex, he told him, 'I hear myself saying, "You won't be able to get it up, you will fail, she will be disappointed, she will leave you for someone else."' The therapist said, 'When I get undressed for sex I hear an orchestra; symbols clash, drums roll, the *William Tell* Overture plays' etc. It was funny but true: you have to take control of the thoughts running through your mind and make them positive. If you hear negative music like the sound of doom as you go into an interview or approach someone to ask them for a job or a date, turn it into *Chariots of Fire* or the theme tune from *Rocky* or anything else that can inspire you. That's what music does: it enhances our moods. The best films play the right music at the right time to lift us, scare us, motivate us or increase our sadness or excitement.

When I got the job on *Celebrity Fit Club USA* I was excited about going to work in America. However, there were a lot of delays with my work visa and every other day an executive from the network would call me in a panic and say, 'What if it doesn't come through in time? What if you don't get it? We will have to replace you. It's a nightmare.' It made me feel uneasy as panic can be contagious, so I changed my feelings by singing the song from *West Side Story*: 'We're gonna live in America, everything's great in America'. I changed it to: 'I'm gonna work in America, it's all working out in America', and hummed it to myself any time things got stressful and any time I felt doubt, so that I was sending signals to my mind that said I feel fine and positive, instead of anxious, panicky and worried, and it all worked out perfectly.

Years ago I was going to a meeting with a major magazine who were interested in featuring and selling my tapes and all the way there I was humming the tune the mouse sang in *Cinderella*: 'You can do it, you can do it, you can really, really do it', because I knew that in doing this I was keeping my mind on how I wanted to be and off how I did not want to be.

Your mind cannot hold conflicting thoughts so while you are

focusing on what you can do you can't focus on what you can't do. While your mind is seeing you succeed it cannot see you failing. It's why many people whistle if they feel a little anxious as it sends a different message to their brains; it's why soldiers going into a war zone often play heavy rock music in their tanks as it psyches them up and makes them excited instead of fearful; it's also why soldiers sing during endurance training to take their mind off the pain. Whenever I have to have an injection I hum something in my head as it takes my mind completely off what is going on and I hardly even feel it.

Find some songs with great positive messages and hum them any time you could be thinking negative or critical thoughts and it will change your state. Some of the best are:

- 'I'm Having the Time of My Life' – Bill Medley and Jennifer Warnes
- 'Make It Happen' – Mariah Carey
- 'Simply the Best' – Tina Turner
- 'We Are the Champions' – Queen
- 'Don't Stop Me Now' – Queen
- 'I Believe I Can Fly' – R. Kelly
- 'It's a Beautiful Day' – U2
- 'Perfect Day' – Lou Reed
- 'Living on a Prayer' – Bon Jovi
- 'Feeling Good' – Nina Simone
- 'Things Can Only Get Better' – D:Ream

How many of the above tunes are used to introduce politicians at political rallies? Ask yourself why. It is of course because of the effect they have and the message they give. Barack Obama used Sam Cooke's 'A Change is Gonna Come' to very powerful effect.

There are countless more so find any song that works for you, adapt the lyrics to your situation so that they silence your inner critic and you will become more confident and more unstoppable every day. Put your favourites on your iPod so you can get your-self into a great state when anything challenging is going on or is coming up.

You Can't Be Replaced

The feeling of being replaced is similar to how we feel when we've been rejected. Our self-esteem can take a huge dive if we feel we have been replaced, especially if we have been replaced at work or in a relationship. It can be a horrible feeling to see your ex happily ensconced with someone else or to see someone in a job that you thought of as yours. Some years ago I worked with a lovely teenage girl called Rachel who had a severe eating disorder, and, while looking at what could have triggered her eating problems, I realised that she felt unimportant. Her father had remarried and had a little daughter who Rachel felt had taken her place. The new daughter was at that age where everyone thought she was delightful and cute and, in comparison, Rachel felt unimportant, unattractive and insignificant. She felt she had been replaced and was worthless.

Realising what was going on, I knew I needed to make her understand that she was irreplaceable so I asked her to imagine she had died and that everyone was standing around her coffin at her funeral. I asked her to tell me how her mother, father, step-mother, sister and friends were reacting to her death. I asked her to describe how each person felt about losing her and what they were saying about how much they missed her. I know this sounds like extreme therapy, but in Rachel's case it absolutely worked. She felt very emotional imagining the pain her absence would cause her family and friends, and began to realise that she could never be replaced. I also asked her father to put out pictures of Rachel in his new house and to remind Rachel that she was every bit as gorgeous as her little sister. So, instead of saying Lucy is so cute at ballet he would say, Lucy is so cute at ballet – she reminds me of you at the same age. Very quickly Rachel's eating disorder disappeared as she understood her issue was not with food; it was with feeling replaced and insignificant.

When my daughter had a hamster it died after two years and we got another, but it was not the same and didn't have the same character as Ruby, her first much loved hamster. We then got a third and fourth hamster but neither was like Ruby. I have had four cats and they have all been unique. At one stage my daughter had two cats, a hamster, two rabbits and a tortoise and they all were unlike each other.

I often talk to clients whose pet has died and they tell me they miss their dog desperately but won't get another one because they are so sure they won't be able to replace it. If we can't replace a hamster or a cat or dog, why would you think you can be so easily replaced? You can't be. It just is not possible.

Because the grave scene was so very successful with Rachel I used it with other clients who had similar issues and it was equally successful each time, which is why I am going to get you to do it too.

Exercise 1

Imagine your life has ended and your friends and family are standing around your grave. Person by person I want you to imagine what they are saying about you, how they are expressing their feelings about losing you and missing you. Really do this even if you don't want to or think it's silly; the payoff will be that you feel irreplaceable and that's a wonderful feeling worth risking feeling silly for.

Once you have done this I want you to stay in your imagined grave and imagine all the things you did not do with your life and all the regrets you have about a life that was unfulfilled and a potential that was not reached. Interestingly, most people don't fear a long life ending; they fear living a life that has no purpose and dying without

---

achieving their goals. You are doing this exercise to rein-force your commitment to make sure this does not happen to you, and to make you determined to do what you need to do to take action and to achieve your goals and potential with the help of all the techniques in this book. Scientific research has proved that when we do written exercises we get much bigger and better results than if we only think the answers in our head. <u>Don't</u> skip the written work: you will get more impressive results from doing it, not thinking it or simply reading it.

STEP 4

Change Your Language, Change Your Life

Study after study has shown that confident people speak a different language to those who lack confidence. Confident people never say things like 'I can't, it's too difficult', or 'I will try', or 'Hopefully', or 'I wish', 'If only', 'It's my dream', 'One day'. They would not dream of saying things like 'I am a loser, I am useless, hopeless, a dead loss, waste of space' etc, so it stands to reason that if you want to be more confident you need to do what naturally confident people naturally do, and one of the quickest and simplest ways to do that is to speak the way confident people speak.

Changing your language is relatively easy. It's a simple step to take but the results you get back are massive. Since words are the structure of our reality it follows that if we change our words we then change our reality. Making changes in the language we use changes very quickly how we feel.

Your mind takes every word you say as literal and accurate, so if you say, 'I can't do that' you are right, whereas if you say, 'I can do that' you are also right. Language and the words you use associated with confidence have a very powerful effect on the body and mind because words have an emotional content, and what we associate with the words we use shapes how we feel about things.

Experiments have been done showing that if we take on someone else's emotional vocabulary we also take on their emotional state. That means that if you copy the language of confident people you will elevate your own confidence. When you use words like scared, pathetic, useless, anxious, depressed, the label or word you use to describe how you feel is the way you will continue to feel. Our mind responds to and loves words that are descriptive because it makes its work easier to do. So now that you know this only use descriptive words that are positive.

We all know that 'we are what we believe' but most of us don't know that, in addition, we are what we speak. Our words become our reality and our brain uses the words we speak to identify what we are feeling. Your brain takes every word you say as literal and accurate, so if you say, 'I am terrified', 'I am petrified', 'I am hopeless', or 'I am useless' your brain will believe you are experiencing terror or hopelessness, and that in turn will increase the fear you are feeling. If you say, 'I am terrified about going for an interview or scared witless about the review I have with my boss' you are dramatically increasing the negative feeling about something that really is not terrifying. It may be uncomfortable or challenging to go for a job interview or review but it is not something that can fill you with terror unless you decide to make it so by using very dramatic language to describe something that is not dramatic at all.

When you use words or expressions like 'petrified' or 'scared out of my skin' you are telling your body you are in a state of extreme fear and your body will respond by increasing the fight or flight response and making more adrenalin to encourage you to run away from the fear. However, since you don't want to run away from your boss or interviewer you can't use the adrenalin coursing through your body and you have made yourself anxious to no purpose. Instead of cranking up levels of anxiety you can turn them right down and even stop them by using words which are much less descriptive and do not make a negative picture: 'I am slightly concerned about the review' or 'I am just a little bothered by the assessment' are much better because they don't give your brain the intense message that saying 'I am terrified' does. Of course you could choose to say, 'I am excited about the interview' or 'looking forward to the review as it's my chance to shine, to show my boss how good I am at my job'. The words you use are your choice and the resulting feelings are also your choice.

Your brain has to accept and act off the words and pictures you give it. Give it less intense words and pictures and you will have a less intense reaction to situations that you previously thought of as stressful. Of course if you give it more intense words you can make the situation more stressful. If you have a tax review or a deadline to meet and you say, 'It's a nightmare, it's overwhelming, it's killing me, it's unbearable' you will have a very intense reaction even before the review begins. If instead you say, 'It's a challenge' or 'It's an issue' you will cope better with it because you are telling yourself that what lies ahead is manageable and that you can cope by the very language you are using.

Don't use words with a strong negative emotional content or words that make a negative picture in your mind because the more descriptive and negative those words are the more they will elevate in a negative way how you feel about the situation.

Whatever we tell ourselves our mind absorbs and accepts. While your mind is used to filtering and sorting information that is presented to you, it has no capacity to reason with the information or signals you tell yourself. It believes whatever you tell it. Because of this, getting into the habit of telling yourself only positive things is extremely effective. You also need to get into the habit of being very aware of the language, the words you use to describe things – most especially to describe yourself – because your mind particularly responds to words and images that are symbolic. The subconscious mind loves descriptive words, words that create an immediate image.

Feeling excited and feeling nervous are very similar feelings. It's only the description that is so very different. If you are scared you feel jittery: your heart pounds and you might sweat a little; if you are excited you may also experience an increased heart rate and increased adrenalin, but the really important thing that will make the difference is the language you are using. We naturally do this at the funfair by going on rides that are scary and called things like Ride of Terror, Wall of Doom or Death Train and deciding to find it all thrilling. When people scream on the rides it is not always possible to tell if they are shrieking with fear, or excitement, or exhilaration precisely because the feelings are so similar. If you are going on a date, or being introduced to your idol, or giving a presentation, or going for your dream job you can choose how you are going to feel by using positive words like excited, psyched, thrilled.

If you use words or expressions like 'terrified', or 'petrified', or 'scared to death' your mind will do everything to stop you doing things that you may actually want to do because your mind will believe you don't want to do them. You can choose to say, 'I feel scared' or you can immediately change this to 'I feel excited. I love this feeling. It's amazing. I feel great' and no one will know that you once felt scared and now you don't, not even your own body.

There is an often quoted story of Bruce Springsteen describing what it was like to perform live. He described it as the most amazing feeling in the world and said, 'When I am performing my heart rate surges, adrenalin flows through me. I sweat and I feel so jazzed. It's better than sex, there is nothing like it, it's the best feeling there is.'

Carly Simon also described what it felt like to perform live and described the same feelings – adrenalin pumping, heart racing, sweating – but she concluded that she was having a panic attack and it forced her to retire from performing live.

I recently got called in to comment on something live on the news and when I got to the studio, as I sat on the stool waiting for the camera to pan in, I thought, 'I really don't want to do this. Why am I here? Why did I agree to this job?' and I knew that I had to change that so I immediately started saying, 'I love doing this, it's such fun, so exciting and I am so good at it', and by telling myself that even though it was at that moment not at all true it made the job a lot easier. You really can choose to be confident by choosing to communicate differently with your mind.

Words tell our mind what we are feeling; the words are the only things that describe our state to ourselves. It's like a bio feedback. If you use negative words you feel negative; if you use positive words you feel positive. We need to use words which are much less descriptive and do not make a negative picture in order to overcome anxiety and fear:

- 'I am terrified' becomes 'I am a little uncomfortable.'
- 'I can't stand it; I can't bear it' becomes 'I can cope', 'I can deal with this.'

Less descriptive words don't give your brain the intense message that saying, 'I am terrified' does. Your brain has to accept and act off the words and pictures you give it. Give it less intense words and pictures and you will have a less intense reaction. Using words like 'It's hell, it's a nightmare, it's driving me mad, I am going out of my mind, up the wall, I am going crazy, this is killing me' makes your situation worse. Saying 'It's bothering me, vexing me, concerning me' causes your body to react in a milder way because the words are milder. Keep your dramatic words and descriptions for things you want to feel: 'I am amazing, it was awesome, thrilling, I am outstanding. I feel phenomenal, I feel fantastic, I feel on top of the world.'

Whatever we tell ourselves our mind absorbs and accepts without question as true, and because of this getting into the habit of telling yourself only positive things is extremely effective. You also need to get into the habit of being very aware of language, the words you use to describe things – most especially to describe yourself – because your mind particularly responds to words and images that are symbolic. The subconscious mind loves descriptive words, words that make an immediate picture.

Here is an example:

A client tells me she has a problem with public speaking and has to give presentations at work, which she dreads. I ask her to tell me more. She responds by saying, 'I'm in pieces; my life is a nightmare because my job is a living hell. I am shattered, I can't cope and I'm a hopeless mess at presentations, I clam up and am frozen with fear when I have to talk to clients.'

So how much of that statement is true?

1. She isn't in pieces.
2. Her life is not hell or a nightmare.
3. She is not shattered.
4. She is not a hopeless mess.
5. She is not frozen with fear when she has to talk to a client.

How much of that statement does her mind believe is true and act upon?

Yes, every single word is accepted by her mind as a fact, and now her mind is working to meet that picture, and because it's such a vivid descriptive picture the mind has an easier job making the picture a reality.

If you say 'I am petrified', or 'It's a nightmare', or 'It's hell' your mind first makes a picture of what that means, and then works to have you feel and act in ways that match the picture you are causing your mind to make. The more vivid and descriptive the picture is the easier it is for your mind and body to act on it. You cannot feel calm, confident and composed while using descriptive words like 'hell' and 'nightmare' to tell yourself what you are feeling. One of the rules of the mind is that your body MUST act in a way that matches your thinking; it literally has no choice. Since thoughts always come first your mind always influences your body and it can never be the other way round. Language is so involved in this. When people are unhappy they use expressions like 'I feel so low', 'I am so down', 'I am sinking', and their physiology is stooped and lowered. When they are happy they use expressions like 'I am so up', 'I am on a high', 'I feel on top of the world', 'I feel brilliant', and their physiology is the direct opposite of someone who is down.

Remember, the way you feel is linked to the way you focus.

And the way you focus is down to only two things:

- The pictures you make in your mind.
- The words you use.

Don't use negative words or pictures. You are not falling apart, peeing your pants or worse at the prospect of going for an interview or meeting a deadline. However, if you keep using words like this you will feel as if you are. You are not having a heart attack and your deadline is not killing you, so stop telling yourself you are. You are not in hell or having a nightmare because you are in traffic or a supermarket queue and your children are not driving you demented and making you pull out your hair.

In order to become confident and self-assured you must banish and forbid talking to yourself like this ever again. There is probably no one in the world you talk to as meanly as you do to yourself. If you spoke to your friends like that they would be long gone. Stop punishing yourself. It is important to remember that criticism withers people and praise builds them up.

Praise yourself more and you will find it easier to change.

Exercise 1

Think of all the words and language you use to describe yourself. Write out all the words then go through them, deciding to delete words that are not positive. As you delete them you can replace each word with a new and more appropriate word, or you can just erase those words from your vocabulary without needing to replace them. Examples: pathetic, stupid, scared, hopeless, useless.

Delete all these words from your self talk for good.

Never say, 'I'm a loser' even if it's only jokingly. Remember, our subconscious mind has no sense of humour and takes everything we say literally.

Now make a list of the negative things you say to yourself similar to the one below then write out and change your statements about yourself and reinforce the change.

NEGATIVE	POSITIVE
I am absolutely terrified	I am calm and in control
I am petrified	I am coping fantastically
I am having a heart attack	I am a little bothered
I am wetting myself	I am mildly concerned
I just can't cope	I know what to do and how to do it
They won't like me	I like me and so do others
I can't do it	I can do it. I will do it. I am doing it brilliantly
I am frozen/paralysed with fear	I am excited and doing a fabulous job
I am falling apart	I am doing so well
I can't bear it, I can't stand it	I can do anything
This is killing me	This is challenging me
My children are driving me mad	I can cope with my children
My other half is driving me up the wall	I can deal with our differences

Once you have written out your new statements I want you to think about how you are going to use them. If you think about new situations as scary just change that to 'It's exciting to have new opportunities'. Remember, the point of this exercise is to give your body the instructions that you want it to respond to. If you hate speaking in public or meeting new people, if you feel anxious before meeting your children's head teacher, just imagine how great it will be to feel that previous beliefs have no power over you and how liberated you will feel when you state 'I can talk to anyone'.

Whatever you have been saying that is negative you can easily flip it over to find the positive that makes a better statement, that helps you instead of hurting you, and choose to say that instead.

I often hear clients saying, 'I've been stuck in the supermarket, it's bedlam in there', or even 'I've had the most torturous time getting here. The traffic is a nightmare.' Then, just for good measure, they will add my back is *killing* me, or I have *starved* myself all week but I still look as *fat as a house*. Without realising it they are using very powerful, descriptive words for events that aren't really that important and need to be forgotten not elevated and remembered in the mind as scenes of hell, bedlam, torture or a nightmare.

If you want to feel confident use words that are very descriptive, that make a picture that is thrilling or exciting and powerful. When I hypnotise clients to give birth I remove the words labour, pain and contractions from the conditioning CD I make for them and instead talk about delivery, birth signals, rushes, feelings, sensations, euphoria. Many of my clients who listen to this during the last stages of pregnancy and during delivery say they love it because it contains no negative words and allows them to experience childbirth in a more manageable way. You may need to persist with changing your language and vocabulary if you have been using powerful words to describe negative sensations for some time. The mind learns by repetition and by the regular process of positive repetitions; using much better language you will see and experience definite changes. Years ago I went on a course in Hawaii that involved walking on burning coals and climbing 50-foot telegraph poles. Before I left England I decided that I would pass on the pole climbing. I stood on the roof of a building that was 50 feet up and didn't like it very much; I noticed that I was saying to myself, 'I'm not going to climb the pole.' When I arrived in Maui and saw other people climbing the poles I declined and said that I didn't want to do it and had no intention of doing it. On my last but one day, I watched a little girl of five climb the pole and this immediately changed my thinking. I decided that if she could do it so could I.

As I changed my thinking everything changed. I began to want to do the climb, and I started to feel excited about it and instead of saying, 'Nothing would make me do it' I was saying, 'I am going to do it, I will do it, I really want to do it.' A few hours later I was standing on top of the pole balancing on one leg having my photograph taken. It was wonderful and thrilling, I loved every moment of it and it was a fantastic lesson to me on changing my thinking and changing my language and feelings. I will always be grateful to that little girl.

Programme Your Mind to Succeed

Just as we must avoid language that is clearly negative in the way that we think and speak, it's important to pay attention to all our language as some words that appear to be harmless and neutral can be negative when used in the wrong way.

For example, 'my' is an ownership word. 'My' is also an emotional word. One of the most forceful rules of the brain is that it is reluctant to give up anything you prefix with MY. The clients I have worked with who had the most anxiety and the least success always talk about MY headaches, MY problems, MY depression, MY illness, MY stupidity. The clients who come to see me to gain confidence would always talk about MY fear, MY anxiety, MY problems, MY nervousness, MY hopeless memory.

This is exactly the kind of language usage that we need to move away from. You mustn't use the word MY as a prefix to something you wish to be free of because this is making the mind accept something as belonging to you when it doesn't. The mind finds it much harder to part with or change anything which you continue to refer to as my/mine. Only prefix something with MY if you are proud of it and want to keep it. For instance, you can talk about MY confidence, MY improved self-esteem, MY commitment to this programme, MY determination, MY enthusiasm, MY fantastic progress in the same way you talk about MY children, MY job, MY car. These are things you are happy about and proud of owning.

We have all seen small children fighting over a toy or even a chair they were sitting in while screaming 'It's MINE'. Adults can get just as upset when someone takes MY seat, MY place, MY newspaper. They become very territorial about something they think they own and your brain is doing the same thing all the time. You just may not have been aware of it before, and now you are it can only help you to succeed in reaching your goals.

Your shyness or lack of direction does not need to be yours. Does it belong to you? Do you call it mine? Do you want to own it for ever, or is the real you underneath. If you say, 'It's mine' and I say, 'I can take it off you', it isn't going to be yours any more. You aren't going to fight me for it, you're going to say, 'Take it all, with pleasure. I don't want it.'

It is pointless and counter-productive to keep calling a habit you don't want MINE while all the time longing to be free of it.

If you don't want it, if you don't want to keep it or own it then constantly referring to it as MINE is giving your brain very confusing messages.

You must prefix anything you want to be free of with the word THE not the word MINE or MY. THE is a neutral word and that's why women hate being called THE wife instead of MY wife as it does not imply pride or connection. It's just ambiguous. As soon as you talk about THE shyness, THE fear, THE procrastination you have no emotion attached to it and it is easier to become and stay free of it. If you slip up, just correct yourself.

You didn't know better before and now that you do you are going to do better all the time.

Even the words you place in front of words will have an effect on how you feel and this is especially true with swear words, which are used to intensify a feeling. If you say it was awful but add in front that it was absolutely awful, bloody awful, positively awful or absolutely f****** awful, you get a stronger response in your mind and body to how awful it was and to how awful you feel it was.

If you say it was amazing then add truly amazing, simply amazing, absolutely amazing, f****** amazing, then you again get a stronger reaction to the event only this reaction is positive where the previous one was negative.

If you describe yourself as an idiot then put in front of it I'm a hopeless idiot or a stupid idiot, your mind creates a much more vivid picture and a more intensified feeling accompanies those words.

'I am confident' is more intense when you say, 'I am *incredibly* confident' or '*constantly* confident' or '*outstandingly* confident'. 'I love taking action' is stronger when you say 'I *always* love taking action'. 'Becoming confident is easy and natural' becomes easier still when you say, 'Becoming confident is *so amazingly* easy and natural.' Swear words are naturally used to increase the intensity of descriptions so use this to your advantage: 'I feel fantastic' is more intense when you say 'I feel fan-bloody-tastic', and 'I am so damn amazing' is more powerful than just amazing. 'Fantastically motivated' is more dynamic than simply so motivated and so on.

Avoid words like Try, Hope, Wish or Dream. Successful people never use these words. They never talk in sentences or phrases like: I am trying to get a better job, I wish I could be promoted, I dream of being in a great relationship, I hope I succeed this time, If only I could assert myself. These words state to your mind that you have no power or ability to make it happen and that you are depending on some external force to make it work.

You are wishing, hoping and dreaming of it working because it is beyond your ability to pull it off. If there is something that you want, don't Wish, Hope, Long for or Dream of it. When you wish for something you send a message to the brain that says, I want this but I don't believe I can ever have it. When you say, I will try, your brain immediately accepts the word try as so insignificant that it does not matter if you get the results or not. When you say *I will* instead you get a very different and positive response.

Saying 'I hope it works' allows your mind to believe that you doubt it will work. Saying 'I dream about success' is interpreted by the mind as dreaming about something because you have already accepted it is not attainable or not going to happen. When you replace the above words with 'I Know', 'I Can', 'I Will', 'I Am', you immediately move into a take-charge-and-succeed mentality. Put those words into your statement so they read like this:

- I will get my promotion (see how *my* works in this situation).
- I absolutely definitely will get my pay rise.
- I can ask x out.
- I know I will succeed.
- I am making things work for me.
- I am fantastic at communicating.
- I know I am a great parent.
- I am regaining the phenomenal confidence and self-esteem I was born with.

When you start to communicate with yourself in this way you are giving yourself confidence to go after things you may have held back from. At first the changes may be subtle and cumulative but as you continue to talk about yourself using more positive language your confidence will become lasting.

How to Know You Are Enough and Have Others Know It Too

'I am ENOUGH' can be the most powerful words of all and are among my favourites. As you work through this chapter you will become aware of just how important these words are and you will learn how to go about using them for maximum impact and lasting confidence.

Knowing that you are enough is such an important aspect of this programme and the realisation that you are enough is a core need. In order to have real inner confidence and lasting self-esteem you must know, feel and believe that you are enough because this realisation is very much at the heart of confidence of all types. Knowing you are enough is so much more than the freedom from needing excessive amounts of material goods. Feeling that you are enough frees you from so many unnecessary insecurities which are impacting your confidence. The feeling of not being good enough, or worthy enough, or interesting enough can be a major contributor or cause of the depression, stress and anxiety that so many people in the Western world suffer with. We feel not interesting enough, not attractive enough, not smart enough, not rich enough and specifically not good enough. Depressed people tend to feel not worthy of help and that they are not worth bothering with. Step 9 covers depression in more detail.

I had been working with people with confidence issues for several years and was very struck by the fact that they never felt they were enough in themselves and often could not get enough: they overspent, overdrank, overate, overcompensated by working too long and too hard, overshopped and often hoarded stuff. It wasn't hard to make a connection and the connection became clearer with every client I saw for therapy for lack of confidence.

Wanting too much stuff and needing to do too much generally stems from an inner feeling of lack, of something missing inside us, or, as one of my patients described to me, a feeling of being empty inside, and therefore we need more food or alcohol, or more material things, or more things to keep us busy, so we can feel worthwhile and compensate for the lack we feel and to fill the void within us. Instead of filling that void with items and purchases or work, you need to understand that the void exists only in your mind and you have the power to close it for ever. One of my clients in America told me she had excessive sickness and at the time I did not realise what she was describing. She was not being excessively sick; she just needed stuff in excess as she felt worthless and empty. Buying lots of items is just a filler for the emptiness. Another of my clients, Emma, was a shopaholic who shopped to fill the emptiness and to feel as significant and valued as she once had at work. Her need to be perfect had made her a workaholic and when she worked herself to a breakdown and had to be signed off, she replaced working with shopping and then suffered dreadful suicidal depression. She became fully cured by realising that she was enough and by reminding herself of this daily. She appeared on *This Morning* discussing her transformation from a depressed and desperate shopaholic to happy, balanced person who had written a book about her experiences and helped many other people. When Eamonn Holmes asked me how I had helped her I told him my philosophy of not being enough and how to counteract it. He interrupted me, and for a minute I thought he was going to dismiss what I'd said, but to my delight he said he believed seven out of ten viewers would relate to that. Emma found happiness and inner peace by telling herself every day that she was enough. I explained to her that everything she was buying was because of how she thought it would make her feel, but she could get the feeling without the purchases. She stopped shopping, paid off her debts, came off antidepressants and started a new business and achieved real happiness. She also shed three stone because she stopped overeating as well. I joked that she went from Giorgio Armani to George at Asda and had never felt better as she has real values and was finally able to like and accept the lovely person she really is.

I cannot emphasise enough how important it is to tell yourself you are enough. It is so simple but the results can be life changing. You must say I AM ENOUGH constantly, say it out loud, say it with feeling, say it like you mean it and say it over and over again and do so for weeks until it sinks in and replaces the feeling that you are not enough which may be holding you back. This will make you feel enough and when you know you are enough you can make eye contact because you don't feel other people are better than you. You hold yourself well, carry yourself well, have confident body language, walk with ease, you talk at the right volume, not loud or soft or fast, you can be heard and you listen and you feel free to have an opinion rather than agreeing with others. You have good energy and as people sense that you feel good about yourself they will like you more. We all gravitate towards people who have integrity. You don't need to pretend you are anything else or to live a lie. You can be truthful about who you are and live in the truth. And the truth is:

- Your past is not you.
- Your bank account is not you.
- Your body is not you.
- Your weight is not you.
- Your age is not you.
- Your job is not you.

These are just the wrappings.

What you look like is just the packaging; who you are inside is much more important. That does not mean it isn't important to make the best of yourself and to ensure that you feel good about how you look, but if looking good made us happy and confident there would not be so very many people who are considered gorgeous who are desperately unhappy and even suicidal.

As you install in yourself a certainty that you are enough you need to remember that some people, who seemed to prefer you the way you were, might be unhappy about your changes, especially if they also lack confidence. We like people who are like us; people who feel inadequate feel comfortable with people who are similar, so your friends or partner or family may resist you changing. You don't have to stay the same to make them happy; if making them happy were to make you unhappy then you could not make them happy. You are Enough, so get into the excellent habit of accepting and liking yourself by beginning and ending every day with the words:

- I am me and I am enough.
- I am always enough.
- I will always be enough.
- I am more than enough.

Make a point of saying these things when you are showering or cleaning your teeth so that as you add one to the other it becomes a permanent daily ritual. Write it on your screen saver, your mirror, stick a note on your wallet and your fridge, write it on your hand if it helps and repeat it to yourself over and over and really get it, because IT'S TRUE!!!! So many clients from my last book have written to me to tell me, '"I am enough" flashes across my screensaver and inspires me every day.'

Many people when they first fall in love totally lose their appetite and can recover from ailments like migraines or skin conditions. During the first flush of love, when they are constantly told by their partner 'I love you, you're amazing, you're the best', they do feel enough, they believe it will be like this for ever and their feelings of inadequacy or their ailments temporarily diminish because they are boosted by someone else's elevated opinion of them. You can elevate your own self-esteem. You don't need someone else to do it for you and by doing it yourself you are not needy – you are self-assured and self-trusting. When we need other people to praise us we are needy and dependent. When we can do it ourselves we are independent and self-assured. We can still enjoy the praise of others but to have true confidence you must praise yourself on a regular basis.

Many people don't understand self-praise, or what I prefer to call statements of truth, because when they repeat a positive statement they come up with all kinds of objections.

It goes something like this.

You say 'I AM ENOUGH' to yourself and you find your mind coming up with all kinds of objections such as:

- I am not really enough because I don't have a great job and I don't earn enough money.
- I am not enough. I don't even have a car.

At this stage many people give up, not realising that it is YOU who is coming up with the objections and YOU who has the power to stop them. To fix that for good, add the objection into the statement like this:

- I may not have a lot of money but I am still enough.
- I am enough with and without a car.
- 'How come I never get promoted?' becomes 'I will get my promotion even sooner as I accept I am enough. As I increase my sense of value and worth so does my boss and my colleagues.'
- 'I am not enough or I wouldn't be alone' becomes 'I am enough and I don't have to be alone.'
- 'How come I don't have a relationship if I am enough?' becomes 'My fears kept people away, but as I accept I am enough so will any person I get involved with. The more I like me the more they will like me.'

It's natural to initially come up with objections to the 'ENOUGH' statements. You simply need to look at the objections and shoot them down with something better. If you keep on with the self-praise and statements of truth, eventually you will run out of objections and your mind will conclude, 'You say this so often and with such conviction it must be true', and with that your mind is agreeing with you and you are finally making real progress.

Now you are becoming a physical expression of what you believe – **I am enough** – instead of becoming a physical expression of the opposite – I am not enough.

STEP 5

Choose Confidence

This probably sounds too simple but you can choose to be confident by choosing to think and behave differently and by choosing to believe different things about yourself. In making these choices you are effectively setting yourself goals, which is so important because human beings are all built as goal-seeking creatures. Our goals give us purpose, focus and direction. Without goals we drift and flounder. Choosing to do the right thing is very good for humans as it makes us move towards our goals. Your subconscious mind is a natural goal-seeking device, so whatever you focus on you move towards and get more of. Your success mechanism is triggered by your goals.

Having a goal and being able to take steps towards achieving it and seeing it through to its accomplishment makes us feel good about ourselves. It can make us feel satisfied, self-confident and self-motivated, more like winners and achievers. The happiest and most successful people are goal-orientated; they are always goal setters. Not only is goal setting extraordinarily powerful, it is also easy if you learn to set your goals in a particular format. There are specific techniques to ensuring you set your goals in a way that takes you towards success; if you do it properly it can change your life. We need to have goals in order to be a success. However, the success is not just in having them; it's in how you design them. The way you design your goals can transform your life and this chapter will show you exactly how to do just that.

In Mark McCormack's book *What They Don't Teach You At Harvard Business School*, the author describes a study conducted between 1979 and 1989. In 1979 the graduating year of a Harvard MBA programme were asked, 'Have you set clear, written goals for your future and made plans to accomplish them?' Only 3 per cent had done that, 13 per cent had goals that were not written out and 84 per cent had no goals at all. Ten years later, in 1989, the class numbers were interviewed. The results showed that the 3 per cent who had clear, written-out goals were earning ten times as much as the other 97 per cent were earning *collectively*. Even the 13 per cent who had unwritten goals were earning twice as much as the 84 per cent who had no goals. That Harvard study was a copy of a study done even earlier, in 1953 at Yale, where again the graduating class were asked a series of questions including did they have clear, specific goals written out with plans to accomplish them. Only 3 per cent had. Twenty years later, in 1973, they went back and interviewed the class members again and found that the 3 per cent that had written goals were worth more financially than the other 97 per cent put together. Not only were they dramatically richer, but they were also happier, better adjusted and more successful at everything they did.

That is the incredible power of goals. Habitually and systematically setting goals improves performance and achievement. You must write out your goals, think about your goals and talk about your goals and make plans to achieve them so your subconscious mind then works to make your goals come to fruition. Current studies still show that less than 3 per cent of people have clear goals and less than 1 per cent ever write them down properly. If you want to be in amongst the top per cent of achievers then do what they do: write out goals the way they write out goals in the specific format contained further along in this chapter.

When you programme your goals into your brain you are moved towards their accomplishment much more easily. Of course, you need to do more than simply write out your goals as if they were a wish list on Amazon. Goals need self-discipline, determination, self-confidence and the self-belief to stay with them until you accomplish them. Don't give up just because they don't work out quite as you imagined or planned; you need tenacity and a desire to keep going and the ability to recognise that a delay is not a denial, it's simply a delay. If you give up when things don't work out you will miss out on extraordinary achievements. Louis Pasteur said, 'Let me tell you the secret that has led me to my goal; my strength today lies solely in my tenacity.'

It's hard to understand why more people aren't taught to set goals and why it is not taught in schools, especially since the schools that have experimented with goal setting find children like it and hugely benefit from it. The pioneer of goal setting is without doubt Brian Tracy. He taught me so much about goals. Brian Tracy states that people don't set goals because:

- They don't understand their importance.
- They don't know how; goal setting is not taught in schools.
- They fear rejection so hold back from goal setting through fear of ridicule or criticism.
- They fear failure without understanding you can't succeed without failure. The only way to fail is failing to try.

It's a common trait for people to fear and resist change in case they become worse off. Goals enable us to control the direction of change in our lives and to ensure the direction of change is towards improvement. It is difficult to successfully control our lives without goals. It's also difficult to feel good about ourselves unless we feel in control of the direction of our lives and of the direction of change in our lives.

One of my patients was very scared of change so instead of pushing her to change I got her to imagine a life without change or risk. First I had her imagine she had a very safe job as a home typist. She lived in a bedsit, she didn't socialise or mix with anyone and never had to risk rejection, but of course in living a life without risk she was not living a life at all. Then I had her imagine she was living in Yemen and had the same life as her grandmothers and great grandmothers; every day the food, the scenery, the weather and everything she wore was exactly the same as it was the day before and it would be the same again the next day. She did not have to imagine her daughter's futures because they would be identical to hers. Then, finally, I had her imagine being in an accident and having to spend the rest of her life bedridden. She did not have to fear change because nothing changed. In doing this she began to link enormous pain to not changing and enormous pleasure to change. I realise this sounds cruel but for her it was so effective that it got her to want what she had feared and to fear what she had been wanting. When I next saw her she said, 'Every time I think about not changing I only have to say the word Yemen to myself and I instantly remember that change is good, necessary and exciting.'

We must welcome change and make it change for the better. That does not mean that it is always easy but fortune favours the brave. As crabs and lobsters grow they eventually become too big for their own shells and they have to make a difficult choice: if they stay in their shell they will suffocate and die, and if they shed their shell they become very vulnerable as they have only a thin membrane that offers them no protection from other predators. Soft-shell crabs have to dig down in the sand and stay there until they have grown another shell (that's why soft-shell crabs are more expensive they are harder to find). So their dilemma is, do I stay in my own shell and suffocate or do I shed it, become vulnerable and then grow? If they are brave enough to become vulnerable before growing we can do the same thing; any time you have doubts remember that if a crab and lobster can do it you can too. **You can't find new horizons while clinging to the shore,** so we must welcome and feel good about change. If you have problems with this, close your eyes and imagine your life never, ever changing. Do that right now.

Exercise 1

Imagine that from today nothing in your life ever changes at all. The weather as it is today is the same every day from now on; whatever you are eating today you eat every day for the rest of your life; whatever you are wearing you wear for the rest of your life. You never get older or change your hairstyle, your job is the same every day, every TV show is the same, you never move home or job, you never go abroad. There are no holidays and there are no weekends. Make this as extreme as you can so that instead of dreading change you dread no change. The reason we love holidays and weekends is because diversity, which means change, is an essential, vital human need. When I lived in LA I loved the rain and found endless hot days became too much as they were all the same.

Doing What You're Good at to Gain Confidence

Why are you here? Not only to find love and have children. As wonderful as that is, you are here to find out what your talents are and to be excellent at something. You can only be good at what you love to do and the key to real confidence and happiness is finding what you love to do and doing it well in a marketable way. It's hard to succeed doing what you hate. Your talents lie directly behind and are absolutely connected to what you love to do. We all have a purpose; you must find out what your passions are and use them, use your gut instinct to guide you instead of being swayed by people who you once might have needed to impress or needed to have like you. Every human has the ability to achieve excellence, to be outstanding in one or more area; everyone is here for a purpose with something valuable to contribute.

Thomas Jefferson said, 'It is neither wealth nor splendour but tranquillity and occupation which give happiness.' That's why we are on the planet – to find out what our talent, our gift, is and to be outstanding at it. You must find your talent or your area of excellence in a marketable skill in order to be outstanding at something that gives you job satisfaction and security – a useful statistic to spur you on is that the top 20 per cent in every field and in every industry will always be employed. Marketable simply means something that you can make a trade out of or something that can be sold, something that you can earn money from. The founders of computer magazines, pet insurance and designer handbag and clothes rentals all found a marketable skill in something they already had a passion for. Anita Roddick founded a global corporation on her passion for ethical products, Lynne Franks founded a hugely successful PR company and then founded SEED – helping women all over the world in business – and has written numerous books, while Jocasta Innes founded a design industry on her passion for paint designs including paint stippling, colour wash, rag-rolling and stencilling. From her passion she founded a chain of shops and has written more than sixty books on paint finish, design and decorating. The new trend for fitness boot camps and military exercise classes in parks is another example of someone finding a marketable skill in a brand new area. Connie Booth, Ruby Wax, John Cleese and Pamela Stephenson have all made a career switch or an additional career out of their interest in therapy.

How well we like ourselves determines how well we do in life. It determines our energy, creativity and response to stress. We can't truly like ourselves unless we know our levels and areas of excellence and we can't find out who we are unless we truly like ourselves. That's why this book is so insistent on you taking on board every step to ensure that you like yourself. We can only be excellent doing what we love to do; find out what you love to do and become excellent at it. What would you do with no need for a wage? What you loved doing between the ages of seven and fourteen is a key to your area of excellence.

Anything significant that you want will require you learning some new skills. So how much do you want confidence and what are you willing to do to be confident? Confident people are confident because they know that they will get what they want. They know they're going to persist and do whatever it takes until they succeed and reach their goals. One of my favourite quotes is 'The lift to success might be out of order but the stairs are always working'. They may have setbacks but they learn from those and do things differently until they get to their goal. They do not allow themselves to give up or hold back. If holding yourself back made you happy you would be happy, but we can't be truly happy if we are not reaching our potential. People who do not realise their potential cannot be fully happy or fulfilled. We don't fear dying, we fear having lived a life without meaning or purpose; we must have purpose or every day is the same, what is known as SSDD – same shit different day. It's depressing when every day is the same as the day before. To make it different you have to feel different inside. Some of the unhappiest people I have ever met are mega-rich, especially heirs and heiresses as they have no purpose and no motivation, and even though they can travel all over the world so that the scenery is different, inside everything is always the same and it all becomes a disappointment because they feel they are disappointing and so, of course, their life is disappointing.

HOW TO SET GOALS FOR SUCCESS . . . AND ACHIEVE THEM

Initially, just pick one goal to work on and then another. Don't even bother with goals such as I want to lose five pounds. Make your goals clear and big and exciting. If your goal is to get more money and you are mistakenly given change in a shop for £20.00

instead of £10.00, you have just achieved your goal of getting more money. But you want more than that – and not because of someone else's oversight! If you want to be noticed, to stand out, and you get a nervous twitch, you will be noticed and you will stand out, but that is not your goal.

Your mind takes everything you say as a command so make your goals absolutely **clear**; make sure there is no room **whatsoever** for **misinterpretation**. Think of it like this. If you went to the hair-dresser and said, 'Cut my hair', but gave them no further instructions, would you get exactly the haircut you wanted? No, of course you would not. If you instructed a decorator to decorate your house or a cleaner to clean your house and left them to it, they would do what they thought you wanted them to but would mis-interpret your desires and move all your stuff and give you a result you were not happy with. So think of your mind as if it is your PA, your secretary or your stylist: let it know exactly what you want and you are far more likely to get exactly what you want.

ACHIEVING YOUR GOALS

- You must have a meaningful goal.
- You must know why you want it.
- You must bring discipline to your goal and let yourself be consumed by it.
- You must be willing to give so much more to your goal than you originally planned to.
- You must believe that you are unstoppable in pursuit of your goal and that achieving it will make you even more unstoppable.
- You must overcome a fear of rejection and go for it (use Step 2 for this).
- You must truly like yourself, love who you are, accept that you are lovable and do every exercise in this book designed to make that happen.

- You must believe you are deserving and worthy of your goal.
- You must be ready to learn new ways of thinking, behaving, talking and reacting.
- You must have faith in yourself and your abilities.
- You must be courageous, take risks (the only risk is not to take the risk); to never take risks is the biggest gamble of all.
- You must create a plan that is *effective* and detailed; and
- You must write it all out clearly.

If you do what you've always done you get what you've always got.

If you want to be different you have to do different and it has to be all the time. You cannot become what you need to be by remaining who you are, so learn some new, specific skill, most especially the ones in this book. When you have completed every exercise up to now then you are ready to set your goals and you are ready to do what you need to do and to become the confident, successful person that you want to become.

STEPS TO ACHIEVING YOUR GOALS

1. Want it. You must want it so very much that the desire for it motivates you to go for your goal. You must want it more than anything and also believe you deserve it and know with unshakeable conviction and absolute certainty that you are entitled to it, that you can make it happen. John McEnroe had a burning desire to win, what he called 'a fire in the belly to succeed'. The industrialist Sir John Harvey-Jones said that the only difference between those who become chairman of the board of a major corporation and those who are merely directors was that the chairmen wanted it more.

2. Believe you will get it. Your goal must be believable and challenging. You must have a fantastic vision of your goals

so that your subconscious mind can work towards it. Goals should challenge and stretch you. Goals will get you out of self-limiting beliefs. Richard Branson had fantastic and innovative ideas for Virgin Atlantic and made it a fantastic airline. Walt Disney had a great vision for Disneyland; he went bankrupt five times before he bought his vision to fruition but he didn't ever give up. He was fired by a newspaper editor in an earlier career because he 'lacked good ideas'. Simon Woodroffe founded YO! Sushi by being a visionary. Sol Kerzner, the billionaire hotelier, said to achieve great success in business you have to have an outrageously rich vision. Successful people have a clear, fantastic vision of their goal.

3. See it. You don't believe it when you see it; you see it when you believe it. Develop a clear mental image; visualise it as if it was already in existence now. This is the most important step: you will achieve it to the degree you are able to see it so make your pictures clear and detailed. If you think you can't visualise, cut out pictures, make a poster, make a story board. Many successful companies put on workshops for their staff showing them how to make a story board in order to help them visualise. A story board is a large board on which you stick pictures and photos of things you most desire, as well as writing on it key messages and motivational, inspiring words. When I wanted to write a bestselling book I did this and when Mark Victor Hanson wanted *Chicken Soup for the Soul* to be a bestseller he cut out the *New York Times* bestseller book list, Tipexed out the number one and typed in *Chicken Soup for the Soul* in its place, then stuck it on his bathroom mirror and looked at it every day. By doing this he was visualising it. The more you visualise the more you believe it is possible. Really successful people visualise all the time. Become more and more clear about what you want. The more you visualise the

more you will believe your visualisation is possible. The more detailed, intense and precise the image, the more rapidly you can achieve it. Make your visualisation big, bright, panoramic and hold its duration for longer. Combining visualisation with intensity of desire increases effectiveness; the more vividly and frequently you visualise the more rapidly your mind responds. When you visualise yourself succeeding you increase your motivation while also unconsciously instructing your subconscious mind to make that picture a reality. The next chapter shows you exactly how to visualise. Visualisation takes practice. What the mind sees it believes; your ability to visualise will have a powerful effect on you. As you visualise you will stimulate your mind and body into action. What you can hold in your mind with confidence you can achieve. We can change our thinking and the mental pictures we make and as we improve them we improve everything. By changing your thinking and your focus, and by making changes in the language you use, you can change your life. Sean Connery always visualised himself making it as a top actor, Whoopi Goldberg visualised herself as a top actress even when others told her she would never make it. When she got an Oscar she held it up and said to the audience, 'Never ever give up on your goals.' Dubai is now a very different and remarkable place because the ruler of Dubai saw how to make it different and hugely successful.

4. Put it on paper. You must write it out. Unless you commit your goal to paper it is only a statement, a wish, a dream. Successful people think on paper. Writing it out makes it real. You can touch it, add to it and alter it. Write it out as a plan; make it detailed in every respect. While you are writing it you are programming it into your subconscious. Make your goals inspiring and empowering and urgent. Venus and Serena Williams have always done this. Write

out how you will benefit from achieving your goals, write out the differences it will make in your life. The more reasons, the more benefits, the deeper the desire = the deeper the intensity of the belief that you will obtain it. The more reasons you have the more the desire and belief that you will have it. The more reasons, the more motivation. DETERMINE WHY YOU WANT IT. Nelson Mandela wanted to be the President of South Africa so he could bring about huge change. He had a huge goal and a huge reason for wanting it and he achieved it. Barack Obama proved that anything is possible with enthusiasm, dedication and belief.

5. JFD is a motto I like: Just F***ing Do It.
   Don't procrastinate. Only 2 per cent do it now; 98 per cent procrastinate.
   The Pareto principle proves that:

- 80 per cent of our results come from 20 per cent of our efforts.
- 80 per cent of our job satisfaction comes from 20 per cent of our work.
- 80 per cent of value is contained in 20 per cent of the things you have to do.
- 80 per cent of your obstacles are internal; only 20 per cent are external.

Everything holding you back is inside you, so do the work, make the calls, ask for help and believe in yourself. Remove internal obstacles by remembering what this book has taught you about not fearing rejection and deleting beliefs that you are not good enough, then keep going.

People who are very successful are not so different from you that you can't become like them. The only real difference between people who succeed and people who fail is that 'people who succeed will do whatever it takes to reach their goals; they will do things they hate if it takes them to their goal', whereas people who fail 'will give up their dreams before they do the things they don't want to do, they won't do the things they hate'. J. K. Rowling wrote *Harry Potter* in a noisy café with her baby in her pushchair as she could not afford to heat her flat. Chris Gardner, the subject of the film *The Pursuit of Happyness*, trained to be a broker while broke, homeless and the sole carer of his little boy. One of my clients trained to be an athlete by running up and down escalators as he could not afford gym membership, and on *Britain's Got Talent* the dance group that came third practised in a bus shelter in all weathers as they had no money to rent a dance studio with mirrors.

6. Join a peer group; find a group of friends or business people who you can share your goals with, set up monthly meetings and commit at each meeting to doing certain things that you MUST have done before the next meeting. Studies show that if you join a group and check in with other people in it for accountability, the likelihood of your succeeding rises from 40 per cent to a massive 95 per cent.

    I joined a wonderful group and committed in front of them to putting on my seminars and because I had made that commitment I put on my first seminars and got my book deal through the seminar. I owe so much to my very own Peer group. We all help each other and they have helped me enormously as without them I may have put things off or delayed them, but once I had told them my plans I could not let them down or lose face with them.

7. Work on your goals daily. The key to huge success is long-term focus on goals. Give yourself deadlines that are measurable so that you can measure your progress. **You can only feel like a winner when moving towards the**

accomplishment of a meaningful goal; happiness is the steps towards your goal as much as its realisation. That's why so many business people who achieve their goals, like the Candy brothers, Alan Sugar and Bill Gates continue to set new ones.

8. Be Decisive. 'Decision' come from the Latin 'to cut off from', so it's important that your decisions cut off the obstacles that can prevent you from achieving your goals. As you write out any obstacles they become smaller when you put them on paper. Think of all the things you regret NOT having done. What stopped you? Did you hold back from talking to someone because you feared being rejected? Did you stop yourself applying for the job you wanted in case you got a no and were disappointed? Have you held back from things because you feel you are too old, you can't afford it, you don't have the time? Can any of these obstacles be overcome or removed? You already know that the fear of being rejected comes from you and is being removed as you work through this programme. As you recall your regrets and identify your obstacles you begin to discover your real aspirations and goals. Danny DeVito was not considered suitable to make it as an actor because of his height. Holly Hunter was considered too small to act as a leading lady, but look where they've got by refusing to recognise obstacles or let them get in the way of their success. Statistically Kate Moss is not tall enough to be a supermodel; statistically at sixty-three Lauren Hutton is too old to be modelling for Mango, which sells clothes for much younger women. These issues have never stopped them going for their goals. Rick Allen, the drummer in the rock band Def Leppard, lost his arm in a car accident but continued to play the drums by using his legs to do some of the drumming work and by designing a customised electronic drum kit. If you think you are too old to pursue

your goals it helps to remember that Frank McCourt wrote the huge and worldwide bestseller *Angela's Ashes* in his mid-sixties after he retired from thirty years of teaching. He went on to win the Pulitzer Prize for *Angela's Ashes* when he was sixty-seven. Mary Wesley had her first novel published at the age of seventy and wrote *The Camomile Lawn* and other major bestsellers in her seventies. She was almost penniless as a widow in her late fifties and did not find success until she was seventy. She then produced a book a year for nearly twenty years and enjoyed huge financial success and critical acclaim. John Mahoney, the actor who played Martin Crane, Frasier's father in *Frasier*, took up acting at forty after becoming depressed and disenchanted with his life as a medical journalist. Buster Merryfield, who played Uncle Albert in *Only Fools and Horses*, worked in a bank for forty years and only became a professional actor at the age of fifty-seven. Roald Dahl achieved his success late in life. Having spent thirty years alone, Anna Massey met and married the love of her life at the age of fifty-three, after a ten-week, whirlwind romance, and is still blissfully happy with her husband, Uri, eighteen years later.

9. Learn something new and expand yourself. Find out what you need to learn to accomplish your goals and learn it. List everything you need to know, pick experts' brains and learn proven success methods from experts. Any goal of significance requires you to learn something new. Oliver Wendell Holmes said, 'Man's mind stretched to a new idea never returns to its original dimensions'. Once you have learnt something new you never go back to your original limitations so everything in this programme that stretches you is expanding your potential and your capabilities. Oprah Winfrey went from being a TV presenter to head of her own show, to owning her own production company, to publisher of her own magazine, to someone who was able

to get a law passed in the Senate, to one of the most powerful and respected women in America today. She came from a humble, impoverished background and had to learn so many new things to get to where she is today.

10. Expand what you do. We enjoy a return in direct proportion to what we give and do to others. Do more; all successful people do more. What you do beyond what was expected of you will determine your success in life. I used to do a lot of work for Marks & Spencer and was impressed that they always did more for their staff to the extent that if I went in after hours they would have trays of cakes and sandwiches left out for the cleaning staff. They always did more in terms of staff benefits and had incredibly happy and loyal staff. The hotels and airlines that I give my business to are always the ones that do more.

11. Be tenacious. Tenacity, stoicism, persistence and determination are vital. The most important goal will not work if you don't work at it, so never quit, never give up. Persistence is a measure of your faith in yourself, your skills and talents and in your ability to succeed. Take massive action every day, focus on the outcome and enjoy the process. The best athletes practise all the time. Someone once told Michael Jordan, the no. 1 basketball player, that he was lucky. He replied, 'You know, the more I practise, the luckier I get.' Gary Player said the same about his skill at golf. Michael Jordan was dropped from his high school basketball team but he did not quit and became the best basketball player in the world. Lance Armstrong didn't allow a brain tumour to stop his goal of winning the Tour de France. Paula Radcliffe describes herself as stubborn, focused and determined from birth. She said that when she is told she can't do something she does everything in her power to do it. Winston Churchill was renowned for his tenacity, his ability

to never, ever quit. Jonathan Aitken, Jeffrey Archer and Martha Stewart did not allow time spent in prison to dent their confidence or their business acumen. Losing out on something, getting a no: these are temporary, but if you give up **you** make it permanent. Many people who were rejected, even laughed out of *Dragons' Den* and told their ideas would never work, have gone on to do very well. In particular Rob Law, who made Trunki, the children's suitcases which are now stocked in John Lewis, was told his idea was worthless. Andrew Gordon, who made the STABLEtables to go under wobbly table legs, was asked 'What are beer mats for?', and Stef Matheou, who made RakaStakas, the plastic strips designed for stacking cans of beer, was told his idea was too specialist. They have all made £500,000 to date. Rachel Lowe, who invented the board game Destination London, was rejected yet her game is selling very well in major stores. **You must come back from no and accept that it is a delay on your way to success, not a refusal that you will be successful.**

12. The other difference that successful people have is that:

- They take action every day in the direction of their goals.
- They begin to enjoy it.
- They delay gratification.
- They do the jobs they hate first.

Studies have shown that winners do the jobs they dislike immediately – making a difficult call, firing someone, going for a run, going to the gym etc. Failures will put off all day the difficult stuff and feel stressed about it all day too.

You can incorporate into your life all the things that truly successful people do, including the way they think, the language they use, the things they believe and even their posture. Confident body language means you walk into a room with a confident, open posture and easily engage with others. Learning from successful, confident people also extends to physical attributes as well as their behaviour or techniques. To adopt the posture of a confident person, always stand with your head up, with a straight back and look people in the eye. Don't mumble, or cover your mouth with your hands when you speak. Behave like this and others will treat you more positively, as someone worthy of their time, interest and respect. If you imagine you have a thread keeping your head up and your back straight it helps, and when you are talking to someone always keep your shoulders, hips, feet and knees facing them. The minute you turn these four body parts away from the person you are talking to you express a need to leave. If you want to appear more interested in someone lean forwards slightly as they speak.

If you are talking to someone and you notice their shoulders or knees or feet starting to point away from you, don't monopolise them. End the conversation and move on or change the subject to regain their interest.

As you continue to work through this book you will absorb more of these techniques until it ceases being what you do and becomes who you are. Studies of very successful people have found that they don't say 'I can' or 'I can't'. Successful people say 'I choose to' or 'I choose not to' instead, and in doing this they are telling their mind that they have a choice, are making the right choice and are happy with the choice they have made. When we stop focusing on what we can or can't do and instead choose to do it, we move away from the denial state and it becomes incredibly easy.

Our mind dictates our behaviour and overrules everything. This chapter shows you how to have a mindset of choice rather than thinking, 'I can't, it's not possible for me', which sends us straight into denial and resistance. As you add your power to choose to your ability to identify and break your patterns of thought and habits, you are beginning a powerful transformation.

Years ago, when I was doing a personal development course in America, I was informed while on the course that part of it in involved skydiving, which I really didn't want to do. I declined the skydiving jump and when they got very American and kept whooping 'You can do it, yes you can – go for it' I got a little vexed (you see, I didn't say I got pissed off, or agitated, or massively uptight – I just got a little vexed) and told them, 'I know I can do it but I am choosing not to. If you gave me a million dollars or maybe even a Porsche I would do it but I don't want to do it, I have no motivation or desire to skydive and I am choosing not to. That is not the same as not being able to.'

When you choose what to do and what not to do you have power and freedom of choice, so if you want to be a success be like successful people and say 'I choose to or choose not to' instead of 'I can or I can't'. Replace the words *I MUST, I HAVE TO*, or *I HAVE GOT NO CHOICE* with I WANT TO, I HAVE CHOSEN TO. It is such a simple change and yet it makes such a big difference.

If you want to work out or get up early and run or do your paperwork, first you have to choose to do it and then you have to choose to feel good about it and convey that to your brain by saying, 'I feel great about this, I love doing this, I want to do it.' If instead you say, 'I hate this', or 'It hurts', or 'It's boring', or 'I don't like it, when can I stop?' you are setting yourself up to fail as the minute we begin to speak in this way our brain begins to look for a way to stop the activity. Saying, 'I am choosing to do this because I am choosing to be successful so I might as well choose to enjoy it' causes any resistance to end.

If you bring work home while telling yourself you hate it, if you go to work early while telling yourself you miss your lie-ins and if you study something while saying this is so boring, you will quickly go back to your old destructive behaviour. Tell yourself you love the freedom to work at home, tell yourself that your body loves early mornings and that studying is exciting as you love learning new things. One of my clients had avoided paying any tax for years and although he came to me with chronic headaches it soon emerged that the cause of them was his anxiety that he would get found out and lose everything. He decided to get an accountant and declare himself and he was so happy and greatly relieved that he didn't get into huge trouble, he did not lose everything and although, of course, he had to pay back taxes, it cost him less financially than he expected. He told me that he loves doing his tax returns now because he no longer lives in fear and whenever he has to pay his yearly tax he chooses to feel good about it by remembering how he used to live in a state of anxiety.

If you hate getting up early, remember what it was like on Christmas morning when you were a kid and could not wait to get up. I could never easily get my daughter up in the morning unless we were going on holiday or it was Christmas, in which case I could not keep her in bed as she woke up and chose to feel thrilled about being awake rather than grumpy. You can choose to feel good about anything at all and you can choose to be confident.

When I was writing my first book I had some resistance to spending my weekends writing. Friends would invite me over and I would say, 'I can't, I have to write my book.' I did not look forward to writing it as it was so solitary. In fact, I was asked to write a book many years earlier and I did not even get the proposal done because I could not face shutting myself away to do it. I kept saying, 'I need to do the writing, I have to do the writing, I must do it' but I put it off and procrastinated because I had not learnt to say, 'I want to do it, I have chosen to do it, I love doing it.'

When I began to say, 'I want to write this weekend' I felt entirely different and motivated. I noticed that I was enjoying the process so much, that one sunny weekend I was sitting alone writing and thinking, 'There is nowhere else I want to be. I am actually enjoying this.'

I hypnotise a lot of students around examination time and I always tell them that they have chosen to study, that for this particular month they want to revise, it is compelling, that they actually enjoy the process, and that it makes them feel so good to do the work. They almost always send in friends who say, 'You hypnotised my friend to study and it's amazing; they are actually enjoying it. Can you do the same for me, please?'

You cannot plan to become more successful and work harder while dreading the process. When I was a personal trainer and teaching boot camp classes I would always get my class to say, 'My body loves this, my body is benefiting from it, my body likes it', and that was true. They may not have liked the fiftieth sit-up but their body really did. If you ran a marathon while telling yourself after the first mile, 'I hate this and I want to go home', you would fail. You could only succeed by telling yourself, 'I can do it, I will do it, I am doing it' because those words would keep you going. When cadets are training in the army they don't bitch and moan about the exercises; they sing and inspire each other to keep going. By singing and joking through endurance training they are sending a very clear signal to their brain that says, 'I have a choice here, I am choosing to do this and choosing to feel good about doing it.' It's the same reason people sometimes sing to themselves when they are doing a tough job as it sends a different message to their brain.

Often simple changes have the most powerful results. Choosing reminds your mind that you have a choice. You can choose to be in control rather than being controlled by your emotions.

By choosing how to communicate with yourself, how to control your thoughts and how to say and think the right things, you really can choose to be confident.

It's essential that you know that you can choose how you feel about anything. As you accept that you can choose to be confident you will understand that every time you say, 'I can't do that, I am too scared, I am useless, hopeless, shy, insecure' etc you are unconsciously choosing to remain stuck and to function way below the phenomenal potential you were born with. As you accept this fact you can also accept that you have not failed at being confident: you simply have not learnt until now how to run your brain. You have been making the wrong choices, using the wrong language and choosing to believe that you just can't help it, but from now on you can choose not to believe that any more. You can learn to be confident, successful and have high self-esteem. It's a process this book is taking you through and re-installing in you.

'Carefully watch your THOUGHTS, for they become your WORDS.
Manage and watch your WORDS, for they will become your ACTIONS.
Consider and judge your ACTIONS, for they have become your HABITS.
Acknowledge and watch your HABITS, for they shall become your VALUES.
Understand and embrace your VALUES, for they become YOUR DESTINY.'

Mahatma Gandhi

'Destiny is not a matter of chance; it is a matter of choice. It is not a thing to be waited for; it is a thing to be achieved.'

William Jennings Bryant

'You are the only person on earth who can use your ability' –
Zig Ziglar

Visualise Your Way to Confidence

In order to be confident you absolutely MUST be able to see yourself as confident. This is not natural or easy for someone who believes they have never experienced confidence (even though we know that isn't true) or who has felt inadequate for a long time, but you can do it with practice. Just taking five minutes a day, every day, to visualise yourself as confident will work.

Scientists in America and Europe have proved that visualisation techniques significantly improve high self-esteem.

When you see yourself as confident you send a clear message to your brain that positively affects and influences your energy levels and your motivation. These changes have a positive impact on your thoughts and feelings which in turn reinforce the mental programming and mind conditioning.

This works because thinking positively about confidence can activate particular neurons in the brain; these neurons secrete hormones such as endogenous opiates, which make us feel good about ourselves.

Negative thoughts have the opposite effect: particular neurons are involved with producing a negative thought and they also produce negative hormones such as cortisol, which is a stress hormone, and stress can lead to anxiety and depression. The brain changes its neural circuitry as our behaviour changes. Studies at Harvard University showed that imagining an activity activates the same parts of the brain as the actual activity. Particular brain cells called mirror neurons are activated just by thinking about an activity, proving again that as far as the brain is concerned it does not always differentiate between what is real and what is imagined.

Remember, habits are merely thoughts and actions that we have learnt and practised. We are not born feeling self-conscious – quite the opposite – or feeling that we aren't worth it; we learnt to believe those things. When you repeat an action you create a neural pathway to your brain that is strengthened with each repetition. This pathway is like a thread that becomes stronger every time you repeat something. When you first learnt to use a computer, drive a car or operate a new mobile phone or any kind of machinery, you had to repeat the actions slowly, but now, due to repetition, they are so embedded in you that they are almost automatic.

When we cease the habit the pathways diminish, the thread shrinks and becomes redundant. I call this rewiring ourselves. We come into the world wired for success and this programme is putting the wiring back as it should be so that you can be the person you were meant to be.

So the key is repetition of these positive visualisations. It takes repeating and practising something twenty-one times over twenty-one days for the brain to create new neurological habit pathways, and in turn it takes twenty-one days for those pathways to begin to diminish if you cease the actions. Research has shown that repeating new patterns of behaviour and thought leads to physical changes in the brain. Various brain studies have shown that it takes the brain a minimum of ten days and a maximum of twenty-one to let go of an old belief and replace it with another one. Twenty-one days of affirmations and new habits of language and beliefs will start to lock in good and positive changes for you. You need to continue the affirmations but eventually this will cease being what you do and become who you are, so it will be almost automatic; and, remember, you will have your audio download to help you even more.

Becoming skilled and adept at visualisation requires you to focus on your new positive images frequently and to use repetition until it is so easy it becomes automatic. Repetition is vital – the more vividly you visualise, the more rapidly your mind and body responds. This is exactly what you do when you drive a car or operate machinery – you visualise the actions you have to take then take them and then the process becomes almost automatic.

Every time you visualise:
- Make the picture exciting and compelling – the brain is at its most powerful when it works with vivid images and pictures.
- Increase the duration and intensity.
- Hold the picture for longer.
- Make it bigger, brighter and clearer.
- Add exciting, positive words.
- Combining visualisation images with intensity of desire while telling yourself you are succeeding will increase the effectiveness.

Visualisation takes practice but remind yourself that what the subconscious mind sees it accepts without question. Your ability to visualise will have a powerful effect on you and as you visualise you will stimulate your mind and body into action. Remember, what you can hold in your mind with confidence you can achieve – athletes who visualise can stimulate all their muscles to perform at a level to meet their visualisation.

Become more clear and detailed about what you want. The more you visualise the more you will believe your visualisation is possible.

Most very successful people visualise all the time. Great actors are by nature very visual: just as they can see themselves playing a psycho or heroine and pull it off, they can see themselves as successful and exuding confidence if it's important to them or the part requires it, and this becomes the image they hold in their mind and move towards.

We can all change our thinking and the mental pictures we make and as we improve them we improve everything. By changing your thinking and your focus, and by making changes to the pictures you form in your mind and the language you use, you can change your confidence, your self-esteem and your life.

HOW TO VISUALISE

If you think you can't do it, that you can't visualise, then you need to be aware that you are already visualising all the time. Every time you say: 'I can't do it, it's impossible for me to speak in public or to someone I am attracted to or in awe of, if I do that I know I will blush, I can't speak up, I can't do interviews, I can't talk to strangers', you are already visualising and it's working, but not to your advantage. You might as well use good visualisations as your mind will believe and act upon whatever you tell it, good or bad. You have nothing to lose apart from your fears and everything to gain by making your words and pictures positive.

Occasionally I come across clients who say to me, 'I am just not visual and I can't visualise at all.' Sometimes I tease them a bit by saying, 'Lucky you, that's amazing, you must never have a day's worry in your life.' When they reply, 'Are you kidding? I worry about everything – my kids, my job, my health', I then ask them, 'But how can you worry if you can't visualise? That's what worry is – visualising about what could go wrong.' We are all visual. Some of us just don't know how visual we are but you do now. You would never find your way home without a map if you were not visual. When you go shopping in the supermarket it's your visualisation skills that take you to familiar aisles on autopilot. When you get a new mobile phone or washing machine, you will refer to the manual several times to remind yourself how it works but with repeated use you become so visual that you will easily use your new machine without referring to the manual at all. If I ask you to describe the layout of your car, the colour of the seats and the style of the dashboard and position of the gear stick and indicators, you first have to visualise – mentally imagine how they look by picturing them – before you can give that information to me. We can all do this.

Many people use self-development techniques to visualise returning an item in a shop or asking for their food to be prepared differently, and see that as an improvement, but then they don't go on to make bigger, better visualisations. Since we can all visualise and get results you must do more, much more, than visualising a free parking place or getting a discount on an item. Don't make one-off visualisations; instead, as you are visualising becoming confident, visualise it as a way of life and see yourself staying confident. Have faith, conviction and unshakeable certainty that you will and you are constantly succeeding and it will happen.

This is to show you the effect visualising has on your body.

Exercise 1

Stand up, take one arm, raise it to shoulder height and, pointing your finger directly out in front of you, begin to turn your arm as far out and behind you as you can. If it's your right arm move it out to the right, if it's your left move it out to the left. When you have moved your arm as far behind you as you can, look behind you and notice where it is. Now return your arm to the beginning position in front of you then close your eyes for a moment and just imagine and see your arm moving even further, up to 25 per cent, behind you. Really see this in your mind for a moment. Now tell yourself your arm is going to move 25 per cent further. Say this to yourself three or four times.

Now open your eyes, repeat the arm moving out behind

---

you procedure and notice just how much further your arm will move.

You are already beginning to see the power of beliefs on the body. As you saw, believed and thought about your arm moving further it did. Do it a few more times to prove to yourself how easy it is to influence your body using your belief system.

Athletes have been using this technique for years, seeing themselves lifting a heavier weight or performing a longer jump, believing they will do it and can do it and then doing exactly that. In fact, many tests have been undertaken proving that in athletics the ability to visualise is equally as important as physical training. When athletes visualise they can cause all their muscles to perform at a level to meet the visualisation. It is now becoming accepted that in the future it is likely that only athletes who use powers of visualisation, as well as training, will succeed because they have an edge and advantage over others.

I recently made a television documentary with some of my clients who are Olympic athletes. They were talking about how many athletes from many different countries at the Olympic Games used the power of thought, belief and visualisation to succeed and how it gave them an advantage over those who didn't and helped them break a world record.

You may have heard stories of people who are slightly built or unfit lifting a heavy object like a car, tree or refrigerator off their child who was trapped underneath, and then wondering how they managed it. In fact, they momentarily saw themselves performing the feat and then performed it because in their mind, in that moment, they believed they could and would do it. You are now ready to believe you can and will become and stay confident, and that you will do what it takes happily and willingly by changing your beliefs, thoughts, actions and language and that you powerfully respond to your good visualisations.

Visualisation is not just about what you see; it's also about what you feel and hear and say and sense. It makes your visualisation more powerful when you activate all your senses as you visualise. The more senses you activate the more real your feeling is that you will and are already accomplishing this, so while you are visualising be sure to:

- FEEL your body as confident and certain.
- FEEL your posture as confident and self-assured.
- HEAR people telling you how interesting you are.
- HEAR people giving you the job you want.
- HEAR yourself on a great date or in a fantastic interview.
- HEAR great news: 'You have been promoted', 'You are hired'.
- SEE yourself radiating confidence.
- SEE yourself with great friends.
- SENSE how very well you are doing.
- SENSE how strong and committed to change you are.
- SENSE that this is the real you and it all feels natural and easy.

At the same time as forming different pictures in your mind you must tell your self different things, just as you did in Step 1 with your attitude and in Step 4 with your language. Eliminate every possible negative word; focus only on what you wish to achieve and move towards. Keep your mind on what you want and off what you don't want. Whatever you focus on you will move towards, so thinking about how you don't want to feel and what you don't want to do simply puts negative words and images back into your mind.

- Tell yourself: 'I feel confident' not 'I am no longer insecure.'
- Think: 'I am taking action every day in the direction of my goals and enjoying the process' or 'I like talking to people, it's easy for me' rather than 'I'm not as shy as I used to be.'

- Visualise, think and say, 'My attitude is fantastic', 'I have high self-esteem' not 'This is easier than I expected.'
- Focus your thoughts positively to 'I feel so committed to this programme; it feels so right' not 'It's not as hard as I thought it would be.'

'No', 'not' and 'don't' are all neutral words in that they don't make a picture and have little effect on the subconscious mind. Thinking 'I am *not* insecure', 'I *don't* feel self-conscious', 'I *don't* feel nervous' causes the mind to lock on to the only descriptive words in the sentence – *nervous, insecure* and *self-conscious.*

If I ask you not to think of a bottle of purple milk, in order not to think of it you have to think of it and see it even though you have never seen a bottle of purple milk before. Try right now not to think of purple milk and you will see what happens: you cannot help thinking about it. By turning over any negative thoughts you will find the positive. The subconscious mind is only in the moment; therefore, when you visualise, create images that are occurring now, this instant.

Example:
- I am becoming more confident and outgoing every day.
- I am calm and self-assured all the time.

Make your words dynamic and descriptive:
- I am confident and successful.

Make it personal:
- **I AM** confident.
- **I LOOK** self-assured.
- **I ALWAYS** speak to other people.
- **I CAN** talk to strangers. I enjoy it.
- **I DO** whatever it takes willingly.
- **I ALWAYS** speak with confidence in a clear, easy way.

- **I TAKE ACTION** every day in the direction of my goals.
- **I NATURALLY DO** what confident people do.

Using the 'I am, I can' technique, add your own words to the following statement or make a completely unique one incorporating changes that are personalised to your own life, so your statement reads something like this:

'I feel so confident about myself. I am at ease around other people. I feel comfortable talking to people. I always take action and go for my goals. It feels great when people pay me compliments, knowing they like me because I like them and myself. I am taking control of my life. As I achieve this I can achieve anything.'

You can add anything that is appropriate and inspiring for you.

To help you visualise your way to achieving confidence, here are some scripts focused on building confidence as well as some specific areas in which you may want to develop, such as public speaking, being impressive at interviews and achieving a loving relationship. You can add your own wording to them or amend them to suit your particular situation, and then you can either memorise them or record them on to a CD or iPod. But even reading them through a few times will have a great effect on you as they will excite your imagination and fill up your mind with positive thoughts, as you imagine how you would look and feel as you radiate confidence carrying yourself with confidence – standing tall, relaxed, happy, open to others and so on. While you see this and focus on this your mind can't see the opposite.

The Script for Confidence

Because you have the desire to have a wonderful life/relationship/job, you develop wonderful, reassuring inner confidence that radiates from you and is reassuring to the people around you. Your confidence is growing daily. You constantly imagine and see yourself speaking calmly and confidently to a group of people. Their focus is directed on you and you enjoy being the centre of attention. People like you and you like them; you find it easy to make friends. You have confidence and poise. You are interested in people and they are interested in you. You listen to people and have a knack of making people feel interesting and happy to be around you; they like you because you are a good and attentive listener. You have a great ability to reach decisions and people know your advice is worth listening to. You have confidence in social situations, you mix with people easily and have fun. You make friends easily because you are genuinely interested in people. Your confidence in yourself grows daily. You like people and you like yourself. You have so many abilities and talents and they are becoming more obvious every day. You believe in yourself and in your ability to achieve success. You can do anything that is necessary for your wellbeing and happiness, because you have perfect confidence in yourself. You can handle any situation you meet. You have confidence in your ability to meet new people and make new friends. People like you because of your confident personality, your warmth and friendliness, you radiate confidence and you have a huge likeability factor. Your personality and likeability are growing daily. Your confidence is growing daily. The most driving part of you, your subconscious mind, is ensuring that you have poise and that you are comfortable, relaxed and at ease on every occasion, as you move on from one fantastic achievement to another. Each day you become more aware of the full, powerful impression these true concepts are having on you, replacing old beliefs with new, powerful ones that are remaining embedded in you and having a powerful, permanent, pervasive impact on you.

Script for Public Speaking

Whenever you need to speak to a group or an audience you do it easily, naturally and with phenomenal confidence. Your voice is clear and confident and people understand what you are saying, your words are always completely and perfectly understood because you define yourself easily. People listen to you; they respect you; you receive a great deal of warmth and appreciation whenever you speak in public. You communicate easily and effectively with good energy. Your excellent mind quickly and cleverly supplies you with a solution and answer to any situation or question. When you speak to other people your voice is clear and strong, your throat is relaxed, your body language is perfect, giving off the message that you are confident, approachable and likeable. Your energy is positive and just right. You make public speaking look natural and easy and for you it is natural and easy; you make eye contact, your voice is at just the right pitch and tone and you remember everything you need to say and say it in an appropriate manner – sometimes serious, sometimes witty, always spot on. You have an impressive talent for improvising, you always and easily think of the right thing to say in any situation, you have a natural talent for expressing your thoughts and ideas in an enthusiastic way that leaves an excellent impression with the people you are speaking to. People listen to you because everything you say makes sense and because your delivery is spot on and leaves a favourable impression with your audience. Each day you become more aware of the full, powerful impression these true concepts are having on you, replacing old beliefs with new, powerful ones, that are remaining embedded in you and having a powerful, permanent, pervasive impact on you.

Sunil came to me to learn to be able to speak in public. He had fainted at his own wedding rehearsal and had a mental block about public speaking. He also hated writing his name and would get anxious if he had to sign a cheque or credit card slip in front of people. It turned out that his father, who had come to Britain as an immigrant, taught him the wrong pronunciation of words so when Sunil had to read in front of the class he pronounced words incorrectly and everyone laughed at him, and he developed a phobia about public speaking which made him insecure. He then developed an anxiety about being judged and would shake when the teacher stood over him as he wrote, which he continued to feel as an adult whenever he had to write in front of anyone. The thought of having to sign the wedding register and give a speech while being watched by a lot of people brought up all his old issues, but in one session they were removed for good. He listened to the recording on public speaking, which is on the audio download and became a different person. He gave a wonderful speech at his wedding and signed his name without giving it a second thought.

This next script is written in a way that can enable you to come across really well at interviews. Many people who are good at driving, fail driving test after driving test because they are not good at being judged and examined. (I mentioned early in the book that our greatest fear is being rejected.) So many people go into situations where they are being assessed and feel tense and anxious because they put too much store on the possibility that they could be rejected. You have already learnt that no one can reject you without your consent and this next script will help you to be self-assured, confident and composed in interviews.

Script for Giving Great Interviews

You are absolutely relaxed and competent in any situation where you are being interviewed or appraised. As you talk to the interviewer or interviewing panel you feel calm, composed and you radiate inner confidence and a self-assurance that your interviewer(s) like and find reassuring. Whenever you are being interviewed you make eye contact; you express yourself easily and you feel confident and positive, your breathing is deep and steady, your body language is positive, your energy is excellent. You know exactly what to say, you always think of just the right word or phrase and you ask and answer questions easily and in an impressive manner. You are professional in every way, dressing appropriately for your interview and doing the necessary preparation so that you can feel even more confident because you know all the information you will need. You feel a wave of appreciation coming from the interviewers to you and you feel at ease around them and equal to them. You can see them smiling at you, nodding in agreement as you speak, encouraging you and being impressed by you. You accept yourself as competent and skilled and suitable for the job. You are totally relaxed, at ease and confident at interviews; you come across as confident and likeable. There is a great pleasure for yourself and your interviewers that you come across as competent and qualified, communicating easily. In any interview you are ready and prepared; you know what to say. You are thoroughly professional in every way, you are so at ease at interviews, reviews and assessments; your level of high self-esteem allows you to express yourself in just the right way. You are so successful at interviews as you have a huge amount of motivation and confidence to achieve your goals. You feel at ease around potential employers and accepted by them; they sense the unique and special qualities you possess which keeps their interest in you. It is easy for you to give an outstanding interview; it's natural because you are talented and you deserve this job so you have faith in yourself and in your abilities. You have the drive, the discipline and the self-belief to achieve your goals and are second to none at this interview. You have the edge. You understand exactly what they are looking for and you deliver it. You surpass your own expectations and those of everyone else and you are far ahead of your competitors. You have continual success at interviews/reviews/assessments. Each day you become more aware of the full, powerful impression these true concepts are having on you, replacing old beliefs with new, powerful ones that are remaining embedded in you and having a powerful, permanent, pervasive impact on you.

Trevor was a city trader who had started at the bottom and could not seem to get promoted, nor could he find any pleasure in his job. He was the youngest son with three elder sisters and by the time he came along his parents were used to the ways of their three girls and did not adapt to his needs. They constantly criticised him for being aggressive and noisy and hard work, while praising his sisters for being quiet and good, until Trevor felt that everything he did was wrong. He was particularly hurt that his father preferred his daughters' behaviour to his son's. We learn what we live and during Trevor's formative years what he learnt was that he was a constant disappointment and that his behaviour irritated his family. Trevor grew up feeling that something was wrong with him and that he wasn't good enough, and because of this he had no success with his career or women until he learnt to recognise that he was a normal, outgoing boy and his parents were not meant to have another girl. They did not appreciate him or recognise his great qualities but he learnt to appreciate himself and to value everything that made him a man. From never having success with women he found his increased confidence and his ease at just being himself, and liking who he was made him very attractive and he soon found a happy relationship. He used the above script for interviews and got a better job with a different bank where he could assume his new identity as a confident, happy, self-assured man where he excelled. He wrote me a lovely letter, telling me, 'People can smell my confidence and I am so happy now that I understand my parents can't ever again make me feel like a disappointment unless I agree with them.'

Relationship Script

As you go deeper into a totally relaxed state you are aware that your strongest desire and your most powerful and compelling motivation is to attract into your life a loving, lasting relationship. We are all programmed to want to share our lives with people we love and who love us. Most people have had problems loving themselves and others but you are free of that now and free to attract a loving relationship with the person who is right for you and who you are right for. Imagine, see and feel yourself having a loving relationship with someone who knows you are lovable, see yourself loving and believing in each other, respecting each other and your relationship and feeling secure about yourself. You can only love another person to the degree that you love yourself and another person can only love you to the degree that they love themselves, so the most vital, essential and crucial step to finding and attracting love is to believe with unshakeable conviction that you are lovable. Every time you listen to this recording or read these words you are becoming more aware that you fully accept yourself as lovable. You easily give love to other people and you easily accept the love that other people have for you. You are filled and nourished by the love that surrounds you now and always and you fill and nourish other people with your love. You know that you are lovable and deserving and worthy of a loving, happy relationship.

From this moment on you are developing a powerful belief in the truth that you always have been lovable and you are lovable now. You accept that your thoughts are a form of energy that radiates out from you and back to people who harmonise with your predominant thinking. Therefore as you know with utter certainty that you are lovable, other people know it too and you are able to be yourself. Revelation breeds intimacy. You attract real, genuine people who you feel comfortable being yourself with, who you can share your feelings with. You are able to communicate and express yourself. You radiate charisma and are easily able to make other people feel good about themselves, which in turn makes them feel good about you. You raise the self-esteem of others and this in turn raises your self-esteem. You are skilled at genuine flattery and charm, you make eye contact and you have innate magnetism that makes you attractive to others. You now find yourself only attracted to the type of person who is right for you. Think of all the qualities you require in the person you want to share your life with. What would this person's qualities, goals and values be? What are your goals, values and qualities that would make you attractive to them? You are ready and able to give and receive love, to be in a happy, secure relationship because you always have been and always will be lovable. You are so much more than your age, your weight or your job title or salary; you are a lovable person and love is all around you, it is available to you and you are attracting it now. Because you are lovable you attract loving, caring people into your life, the more love you give the more you get back and the more you have. You are lovable and you have a loving, happy relationship. Each day you become more aware of the full, powerful impression these true concepts are having on you, replacing old beliefs with new, powerful ones that are remaining embedded in you and having a powerful, permanent, pervasive impact on you.

Script for Calmness and High Self-Esteem

As you go deeper into a totally relaxed state, you are aware of a wonderful transformation taking place in your personality. You are constantly growing and realising a new sense of self-confidence. You are aware of a new freedom to like yourself; you expect and find that people like you. Your judgement is good and you make the right decisions. You like yourself and others like you. You do good things for yourself and you enjoy doing good things for others. You believe in yourself more every day. You are learning to act with unlimited confidence and high self-esteem because you are using the wisdom and energy of your subconscious mind. You are directing your life and you know life is bringing so many good things to you. You feel warm and friendly when you meet people and they return this warmth to you. Your smile and your friendly feelings draw people to you. You radiate confidence when you meet people. You have perfect confidence that you can handle any situation you meet. You are secure within yourself, confident and self-assured. You deserve the best life has to offer, and you use your inner resources to get the things you want. You are poised and you speak confidently and with a steady, strong voice. You are unique in that you are the only person exactly like YOU, and life has a good reason to express itself through you. You like people and people like you. They like you because you are confident and strong and because you express yourself clearly. Each day you become more secure and more comfortable giving and receiving love. You are a happy, confident person and you like and respect yourself. People like you and give you their friendship because you are worthy of it. You are discovering so many talents that are emerging from your subconscious and you are letting your imagination work for you. Every day you feel more confident that you can handle and solve any issue life has to offer, because you are a good, lovable person and you think clearly and act positively. You have poise, confidence, high self-esteem and fantastic ability. Each day you become more aware of the full, powerful impression these true concepts are having on you, replacing old beliefs with new, powerful ones that are remaining embedded in you and having a powerful, permanent, pervasive impact on you.

As you read or listen to your visualisation scripts over and over again, you may notice immediate or more subtle changes. Change can be retroactive in that it's only later that you realise how much you have changed for the better. It can also be cumulative in that you notice changes on an ongoing basis and for some people it is immediate and very noticeable. You will change on your own timetable so don't compare your changes to those of others. It's a bit like learning to drive: some people have lessons and pass their test first time; others don't; but once you have your driving licence you are equal to everyone else who has one and it no longer matters how many lessons or tests it took to acquire it. As you use the scripts you may need to adapt them to suit your changing needs. For instance, after you have got the job you wanted you may adapt the script to getting a promotion or getting more responsibility within the company. After you have found a great relationship adapt the scripts so you communicate well and make it work and continue to feel lovable and loving.

STEP 7

- Confidence in your feelings.
- Confidence in your relationships.
- Confidence in your needs.

Confidence in Your Feelings

Triple A means being:
- **AWARE** of your feelings.
- **ACCEPTING** your feelings.
- **ARTICULATING** or **ASSERTING** your feelings.

Your feelings are the most real thing you have; they are there to give you a message and you should always be aware of what your feelings are trying to tell you. Many people don't even get to the first A; they are so out of touch with what they are feeling that if they feel something they don't like they have a drink or eat something or shop or make a phone call – anything but feel the feeling. To be at peace with yourself and to have confidence and high self-esteem you MUST become fully Aware of what you are feeling. **You can only be at peace with yourself if you are honest with yourself about what you are feeling.**

In order to do this, don't question WHY you are feeling what you are feeling or try to deny it. Just Accept what you are feeling, even if it is anger, or jealousy, or resentment. If you deny what you are feeling it will just get stronger; the feeling is trying to tell you something so accept it, whatever it is.

Finally, you must Articulate, verbalise out loud and Assert what you are feeling. You don't need to say it out loud to your boss, relative or friend, even if they are the cause of your feelings, but you do need to say it, even if that means locking yourself in the car and saying, 'My sister-in-law/boss/neighbour is annoying, irritating, mean, unreasonable.' Many people make themselves unhappy by telling themselves they can't accept their feelings and they can't change them, so they just go round in circles feeling worse. By being aware of and accepting your feelings as well as asserting them you will become free of this situation.

- Expressing hurt is essential and crucial to our wellbeing.
- When you become aware of your feelings you are already more evolved and sorted.
- When you accept your feelings you are already at peace with yourself, which means you can like yourself more.
- When you verbalise/articulate the feelings you are emotionally free.

Many people have fantasy arguments in their head because they don't express their feelings when they need to. The fantasy is the need to express the feelings; it is internalised anger that we use to play out scenarios in our head where we say what we feel and get the better of people who don't appear to care about our feelings.

It is so important to live in the moment. It's all we have. The future isn't here and the past is gone, so live in the moment by feeling the feelings of the moment, which are joy, hurt, anxiety and anger. You can only express anger in the moment. If you wait and hold on to it, only to express it years later, it will never give you satisfaction because others won't recall it as you did. The definition of madness is the length of time it takes to express your anger over a hurt. You can't tell your partner twenty years later that he bought you the wrong gift or that he favoured his family over you, or tell your parents that they favoured your sister or sent you to the wrong school as their memory of it will no longer be accurate, so get used to expressing your hurt as close to it occurring as possible, out loud to the person who caused the hurt or out loud to yourself – it's still amazingly effective – or by email, letter or text if that helps you.

Don't accuse and say, 'You made me, you hurt me, you upset me, you didn't, should have, forgot to.' Instead say: 'I was hurt when, I FELT HURT BY, it hurt my feelings when', so you are not accusing them, you are simply telling them how you felt when ——————————.

PRACTISE PPP

For a problem to really be a problem it has to be:

- PERMANENT
- PERSONAL
- PERVASIVE

Look at the issues in your life. Your boss is irritating. That is not permanent; in fifteen years' time you will both be somewhere else. It's not pervasive because he/she is not in your life when you are on holiday or at weekends. It's not even personal. He is short-tempered with everyone.

Your teenager is messy, rude, disrespectful and ungrateful and thinks you have the words 'cash dispenser' printed on your forehead (yes, I have one of those too. How did you guess?). They are not going to be teenagers permanently. It's not pervasive as teenagers spend a lot of time in their room or out of the house since their parents are so particularly irritating and annoying. It's not even personal; they find all adults dull, out of touch and boring.

Using PPP will allow you to feel more in control of your situation and more confident. If your problem is not permanent, pervasive and personal it's not really a problem. It's something temporary that you can deal with.

ANGER IS NOT BAD, IT'S GOOD

Everyone feels anger; even newborns and tiny kittens and puppies express anger. Anger is an important feeling and it is there to protect you. Anger only becomes dangerous when it is not allowed to be expressed and so pent-up, unexpressed anger becomes rage or outrage (rage coming out). Not expressing anger can cause as many problems as expressing it too much.

- Pain in the past is anger.
- Pain in the present is hurt.

All anger covers hurt. When you feel angry it's essential to ask yourself what hurt has caused the anger as there is always a hurt behind anger.

So the key if you feel angry is to understand and accept that you have been hurt and then acknowledge the hurt that you are feeling and express it. Be aware of and accept you have been hurt and express the hurt; choose to be honest about your feelings. I really had to make myself do this and it wasn't easy, nor did it feel natural the first time I called someone to tell them how hurt I was by their behaviour, but the results I got back were so good I made it a way of life until it stopped being what I did and became a part of who I was. Even if you don't always get back the results you expect you will still feel better about yourself whenever you express your hurt because you are doing this to give yourself inner peace and confidence, not to make the other person apologise, shape up or feel bad about themself.

When you don't express your hurt as you feel it, the hurt gets internalised as anger and when it becomes anger it joins up with other anger until you have a well of rage within you which will leak out at any opportunity. Someone cuts in front of you on the road or in the supermarket and you explode and overreact. That anger is not about them, it's about old stuff; it's like putting chicken pieces into your freezer in individual portions and then getting them out and finding they are all frozen into one big lump and you can't separate them. Anger loses its label over time and becomes one big lump of rage that the body uses every opportunity to get out. Someone interrupts you and instead of you saying, 'You just interrupted me, I had not finished speaking' you lose your self-control and scream because your body uses every angry outburst as a chance to leak out some of the old stored-up anger that has nowhere to go and really wants to be expressed. Deal with your hurt as it occurs and you won't need to be in this situation. You cannot be confident while you are full of anger as it eats away at your self-esteem, and when people lose it and scream at someone they rarely feel good about it afterwards. Of course, you can still express annoyance and frustration but shouting about it never helps. The calmer and more logical you are as you express annoyance the better results you will get back.

When you are in pain you can say this hurts or that hurts. The absolute key to inner peace and happiness is expressing your hurt as close to the event as possible. The definition of madness is how long it takes to express hurt. When my daughter was little she banged her head and I began to say, 'It's okay, don't cry' and she said, 'Mummy, I am crying because it hurts.' I learnt when she hurt herself to say, 'Ow, that really hurt, didn't it. Poor you', and she preferred that as she needed to express her hurt not pretend it was not occurring. I learnt so much from her and got much better about telling someone they had hurt my feelings rather than pretending it was okay when it wasn't. In relationships it's very common to NOT express your feelings, to hold it all in. It is very bad for your emotional wellbeing to hold on to hurt or angry feelings. That's why I designed the exercises in Steps 2 and 3, and as long as you did them correctly you will have moved on from this now. When I was training as a therapist my amazing teacher always told me, 'Tell the truth about what you're feeling. Be honest. It is the best thing you can do.'

Now that you know what to do with your own feelings and how to accept them and express them in a better way, it's time to do some work on the feelings of other people in your life. No matter how skilled you may become at expressing yourself you also need to understand other people's feelings. Once you can confidently address the issues in your life and deal with them constructively in your relationships, you will find that your confidence grows because you are successfully communicating and successfully resolving situations in a way that is sensitive to others as well as achieving results that benefit you. This in itself will give you a massive confidence boost.

Confidence in Your Relationships

We all need to have relationships and not just with a significant other, but with friends, family, colleagues and other people. The key to successful relationships is how well we communicate and how effectively we meet the needs of the important people in our lives and how well they meet our needs. It is a fact that if you meet other people's needs they will never leave you. However, you may wish to leave them if your needs also are not met. When you are confident you will be a better communicator, which means you will have better relationships, and when your relationships are good they will enhance your confidence so it is a win-win situation. The better you are at communicating constructively the easier it will be for you to get on with people at all levels and enjoy great friendships and intimacy. When you have high self-esteem you feel worthy of getting your needs met and when you have low self-esteem you don't feel that you or your needs are worth meeting. As your self-esteem grows you will feel more worthy of asking for the things that are essential in good relationships such as time, support, respect and being listened to.

No matter how successful you become and how confident you are, it won't mean enough if you don't share your life with other people. The most successful people in the world all state that relationships and family are crucial to their wellbeing, their confidence and their happiness. No one on their deathbed says, 'I wish I had spent more time at work; if only I had chaired more meetings. I regret not having a second car; if only my home was tidier.' They regret not spending enough time with the people they love or not having enough love in their lives. We need to be loved but no one teaches us how to have superior relationships, so in this chapter I am going to take you through some steps that will enable you to communicate more successfully in your relationships to get the most out of them, which in turn will increase your confidence. It has been said that the key to successful relationships is how you communicate. The better your communication and listening skills the better will be your relationships and your confidence. You can't share your life with another person and never argue but you can learn to argue in a way that is more productive.

If you remember the Pareto principle I mentioned in Step 5:

- 80 per cent of your results will come from 20 per cent of your efforts.
- 80 per cent of your happiness will come from 20 per cent of your experiences.

This means that by putting in an effort to listen more, to communicate better and to be more understanding you will get back eight times the effort you put in. Knowing this means that you don't have to view working at your relationship as hard work but as something that will give you huge rewards for smarter effort rather than sustained effort.

There is nothing like coming home to people who love you and are loved by you. When people love and care for the real you, it bolsters and enhances your confidence. I can remember a time when I was in hospital and all my friends came to see me and stayed in my room before and during my operation. They were still there when I came back from surgery and I felt so loved and cared about. It made a horrible situation positive and I will always remember how I felt on that day because I knew they cared about me. Interacting with people in a loving, nurturing way is like watching your child grow and develop and knowing that you helped shape them. Having a positive impact on someone else, being an influence and a driver towards the positive in a relationship is very empowering and rewarding, and there are ten steps you can take to ensure you get the best out of relationships.

We all have the same needs and overall, as I said before, our greatest need is to be accepted and not rejected, because then we are secure in our relationships. Feeling secure is a need. We also have other needs and as we meet our needs we grow in confidence and self-esteem. In the same way that small children don't whine or act clingy and insecure when they know their needs will be met, you will be more secure, self-assured and confident as you recognise your needs and can meet them. We all have a need to be *admired and appreciated* and many of us have a need to feel *valued and desired*. Worldwide, our greatest fear is rejection and our greatest need is acceptance; that's why rejecting our partner's behaviour, looks or achievements is so personal, whereas saying, 'I love you even though you are so moody' feels like complete acceptance. As you increase your own confidence it will have a beneficial effect on the confidence of your family members.

Just as you have needs in a relationship, so does the other party in the relationship. As well as helping them understand your needs, to maintain a great relationship you must recognise and meet some of your own needs and your partner's. The basis for a successful and enduring relationship is to find out your partner's needs and meet them.

Women in particular have a belief that the right man will know what to do (especially in the bedroom), what to say and what gifts to buy. Your partner is not psychic and cannot meet your needs unless you say what they are. The other essential elements of a good relationship are honesty, commitment, time and reciprocity. The classic signs of a relationship in trouble are resistance, rejection, resentment and repression. When a relationship is not working out there are some very clear signals to pay attention to, including withdrawing, 'throwing up the hands in an appeal to God gesture', which means I can't deal with this, and pursuing the other person in the face of withdrawal. You can repair and rejuvenate a relationship by looking at the ten ways that threaten and can end relationships and choosing to change your behaviour. No one can fix what they don't understand but when you understand what may be causing your relationship to flounder you have all the tools you need to fix it and end behaviours that are counter-productive.

Remember, if you do what you have always done you get what you have always got. If you want different you have to do different and it has to be all the time or at least almost all the time, not just some of the time or whenever you remember.

Ten Things that Threaten Relationships

Below are the ten most common things that threaten and damage our relationships. By avoiding doing them you will have better relationships, which in turn will make you feel better and more confident about yourself.

1. STOPPING STONEWALLING

Stonewalling means when one partner refuses to discuss issues or refuses to respond to complaints or requests and says:

- I won't discuss it.
- I'm not talking about it.
- Get over it.
- Whatever.
- I don't care.
- I'm just not interested.
- That's too bad.
- Talk to the hand because I'm not listening.
- Blah blah blah.

Stonewalling is failing to pay attention to your partner. We all need to be heard and, remember, I said in Step 1 that our greatest fear is being rejected so don't reject someone by refusing to listen to them. You can listen without having to respond or you can say, 'I can listen to you but I need some time to respond', or you can say, 'Can we discuss this tonight over dinner as I can't give you the attention you need right now?' Make an effort to avoid dismissing the feelings and needs of others. Even if what they're saying is annoying or unimportant to you, it's incredibly important to show others that you are taking on board what they're saying to you.

2. AVOIDING CONTEMPT, SCORN, MOCKERY, SUPERIORITY

Contempt and mockery are two of the most destructive elements in a relationship and among the hardest things to recover from as they are so personal. Verbal contempt and mockery are the worst but mocking and being superior with body language is also very damaging, such as rolling your eyes, grimacing or sighing deeply when your partner or relative tells a joke. If we believe in the idea that our confidence is affected by the way others treat us, it's just as important to work on the way we treat others. One of the quickest ways to raise your own self-esteem is to raise the self-esteem of others.

3.   DON'T DO DESTRUCTIVE CRITICISM

Criticise your child or partner's behaviour, not your partner themself.

It helps to remember we are not our behaviour.

A good person does bad things sometimes and a smart person does stupid things sometimes too. Destructive criticism is saying things like:

- You are so stupid to forget to bring the map.
- I can't believe how dumb you were not to call first.
- You idiot, you have got lost/gone in the wrong direction.
- You didn't pay the bill on time. You are useless/hopeless.
- You have not left enough time to do this/get there, you loser.
- You left the oven on all day, airhead.

Criticise only the act:

- You didn't pay the bill on time.
- We needed the map to get there.
- You agreed to call ahead first.
- You did not leave anything like enough time.
- When you left the oven on it could have caused a fire.

I taught my daughter this when she was small. I would tell her she was a good girl but did naughty things rather than call her bad or stupid.

If I asked her why she spilt juice all over the floor she would reply, 'Because I am naughty' and I said, 'No, you're a good girl but you did something naughty. Why?' Then she would say, 'Well, I wasn't looking while I was walking with the juice.' So she learnt something without it affecting her self-image or self-esteem, so it was constructive criticism not destructive criticism. I knew it was working when I was late to collect her from school and her teacher said, 'I have just been put in my place by a five-year-old. I said to her, "Your mother is hopeless" and she replied, "My mummy is not hopeless, she's just late."'

You have every right to criticise behaviour and to tell your partner how you feel when they are late, forgetful or unkind, but don't call them names. Constructive criticism helps development and destructive criticism withers people's spirit, whereas praise helps them to grow and is a fantastic confidence booster. When your children play up it's much better to say, 'This isn't you, it's not like you to be like this, what is going on?' rather than say, 'Why are you such a horrible bully to your sister?' Don't feel you have to become a saint and get this right all the time. I never have and I teach this, but even doing this half the time will improve your relationships and your confidence as well as the self-esteem of the people you love. Remember, superior people praise. Inferior people criticise all the time. People who are overtly critical always have the most criticism for themselves and reflect it out to every-one else in order to elevate themselves and diminish others. It is also very important to remember that you have a relationship with yourself so don't use destructive and negative criticism on yourself along the lines of 'I ALWAYS mess things up, I NEVER get things right, I am stupid, hopeless, useless, an idiot' etc.

4. STEERING CLEAR OF HITTING BELOW THE BELT

This is when you use a partner or loved one's weakness, illness, infertility, disability, lower income or status or their past to win an argument, to score points to make them feel inferior and you superior. Saying things like 'Well, no one in *my* family is divorced', '*You* are the one who's too old to have children', 'We can never make plans because of *your* migraines', 'I put more money into our home than *you* do', 'It's *your* family that have caused this mess' is verbally attacking the other. Hitting below the belt badly affects the confidence and the security of the person you are attacking. I have worked with so many families who have a mix of his children, her children and their children. They seem to have the greatest problems when they view the children as yours, mine and ours; when they can see all the children as our children and all the relatives as our family or our relatives it makes them united instead of divided.

5. AVOIDING DEFENSIVENESS

This is when someone does not take responsibility for their actions but instead says, 'It was your fault, you made me do it.' Responsibility literally means an ability to respond. If you can't say, 'Yes, I handled that really badly and I am sorry' then you can't expect anyone else to either. We like people who have the courage and confidence to say 'I was wrong' because we recognise it takes courage and confidence to do that, so they go up in our estimation, whereas people who will never accept they were wrong tend to be alone as they are very hard to live with. You will set a great example to the people you interact with when you can do this.

Don't say things like:

- You made me do it.
- You drove me to it.
- It was your fault.
- You caused this to happen.

And remember: no one can make you do or feel anything unless you let them.

6. STOPPING REFERENCES TO THE PAST AND TO PAST WRONGDOINGS

We can never undo the past and constantly referring to it is counter-productive and leaves the person who was in the wrong still in the wrong years later, so this relationship is out of balance with the wronged and the wrongdoer still playing old parts. For the person who was wronged they believe they get a lot of mileage from being right. In order to be right someone else always has to be wrong. It is much more important to do the right thing than it is to be right.

It's more important to be kind than it is to be right. Interestingly, studies have shown that when a person who commits suicide leaves a note they frequently mention being made wrong and how hard it is to live with that. People who are always right often end up alone because they cannot compromise, so it's a habit of behaviour we all need to avoid, even if we've been badly wronged by someone. Most of us hate to be made wrong and you do not need to make your partner wrong in order to resolve an argument. Talk without going over the past. Remember: you're having an argument not a history lesson.

If a partner has had an affair the other partner must feel that they are allowed to talk through it and to get answers, but not indefinitely. What I find works is to allow the other partner a time period, decided by both partners, when questions will be asked and answered, the issue will be dealt with and then a cut-off point will come when the issue is put away. My partner once said to me, 'You know, you and I are going to have to find something new to fight about because this issue is becoming closed and we don't need to discuss it any more.' It was good advice. It was not stonewalling. We had exhausted the issue and it was time to close it and move on. The key is to close it down effectively and by mutual agreement.

To be happy and have inner peace we must be able to forgive the past, live in the present and feel excited about the future. You can't live in the moment if your arguments are history lessons about the past. If you find it hard to do this go back to Step 2 and do the exercises designed to allow you to let go and move on. You can say all the things you needed to say even if the person is not in the room. You can't forgive the past and move on until you can let go of old hurts and resentments. It is essential to express hurt. One of the keys to having emotional wellbeing and inner peace is being able to express our hurt as close as possible to when the hurt occurred. One of the ways madness is defined is the length of time it takes unbalanced people to express their hurt.

If you keep going over an old argument you may have never really expressed your hurt, so do it properly. Say 'I was hurt by —— and I was hurt when ——', then you can move on. Use the exercises in Step 2 to make sure you do this fully and in a way that works.

Another definition of madness is doing the same thing over and over again while expecting a different result. If you do what you have always done you get what you have always got. If you want a different relationship you have to do things differently.

To have a healthy relationship each partner must have the self-confidence and awareness that they are allowed to express their hurt and to discuss the situation. But there absolutely must be a cut-off point where the issue is dealt with and put away/left behind so that the relationship can move on.

Both partners must agree to this.

- Don't make your argument a history lesson.
- Stay in the present all the time.

You are arguing to resolve an issue not to get even, or get revenge, or even to win. Remember: for you to win the other person has to lose.

We can get upset when our partner wants to have sex after a fight and women often tell me their partner is insensitive, wanting to have sex after they have shouted at them or said some hurtful things.

Human beings have a need for connection and men like to reconnect with their partners through sex. It is one of nature's ironies that women need intimacy in order to feel sexual whereas men need sex in order to feel intimacy. If you are in this situation look at what your partner is intending. Maybe they truly want to connect with you and this is the way that works for them or makes sense to them. If you look at the intention rather than the words or actions you will be much more sensitive to your partner and more in tune with them. Men want to have sex to connect and to make up not because they are selfish or insensitive; they are very solution-orientated and to them it is a solution.

7. UNDERSTANDING THE DAMAGE FROM THREATENING TO LEAVE/END THE RELATIONSHIP

Would you threaten to leave your children when they annoy you? Security is a need and in relationships we need to feel secure. The most secure relationships are those where the partners agree they are staying together and working it out, not threatening to leave. The minute you threaten to leave you devalue the relationship; you have a negative effect on the other person's confidence and if you threaten to leave often it will have no power any way, which will lessen your confidence. I have worked with so many clients deeply damaged as children because one parent would threaten to leave when things got tough. Sometimes they even went through a ritual of putting on their coat, picking up a bag and walking off, leaving deeply traumatised children behind who had no idea it was an act designed to make the other partner shape up. It never works. The more you threaten to leave the less secure your relationship and partner will be, and if you or your partner are insecure your relationship will be less happy because you cannot be confident while insecure. You will grow in confidence and inner security when you know you can work things out. Many people who do leave relationships when they hit a difficult patch just go through the same situation with their next partner, and they never really learn the invaluable skills of sticking with someone through a rocky patch and growing a really stable, secure, loving relationship.

8. AVOIDING THE WRONG ROLES IN RELATIONSHIPS

Many couples descend into a parent/child relationship where one partner is the critical, bossy, nagging or controlling, punishing parent and the other is the child who is always wrong, always in trouble and always expected to improve, to come up to scratch and to stop disappointing the other. Knowing your partner is frequently disappointed in you, by you or with you is demoralising, eats away at your confidence and causes sex to end. We can't have sex with someone who reminds us of our parent. Nature turns off our sex drive in this case as it feels so wrong, incestuous and unnatural.

Many couples lose their intimacy and desire when they have children. They can become so consumed with being good parents that they lose themselves. If we start to see our partner as a parent rather than our partner we don't feel the same physical attraction. Men can never have sex with Mummy and women make a huge mistake when they mother their partners in a caring or nagging way as it destroys intimacy. Women quickly lose physical attraction for a partner who becomes like a father figure by being controlling, dominant, withholding and always right.

Unhappy couples focus on the negative rather than the positive.

Don't focus on what you don't like about each other because whatever you focus on you feel and get more of. Remembering what you fell in love with and how you used to feel is more effective at reactivating those feelings. Talk with each other about why you got married, what you liked, admired and loved in the other person.

To stay in love you must engage in:

- Holding hands
- Touching
- Deep listening
- Stroking
- Shared humour
- Warm voice
- Appreciation

Within a year of marriage saying 'I love you' drops by 44 per cent, compliments and approval drop by 30 per cent, doing something nice for your partner drops by 28 per cent and shared physical affection drops by 39 per cent. Now that you can see these figures you can make sure your percentage goes up again not down.

If we are not part of the solution then we are part of the problem; instead of focusing on the problem focus on how to fix it. Think of five new things you can do to improve your relationship. This immediately moves you forward. A common relationship mistake is to wait for the other person to do what you want and to give you what you want before you respond to them. A successful relationship involves each partner giving 100 per cent. Give what you most want to get back and don't wait for your partner to do the same before you begin. If you give your partner what you know they need the most it makes it easier for them to do the same for you.

- The no. 1 issue couples row over is money even when they are very rich.
- The no. 2 issue is the division of household chores.

Couples fight over money even when they are rich and have no money worries. With arguments over the division of chores, only being faithful and a good sex life score higher than sharing chores on a list of things that make a relationship happy. Research shows that women usually take on about two-thirds of the household chores, while men usually do more external work like the garden, car washing, taking out the bins etc.

The process of dividing the chores is based on your tolerance for mess and untidiness. If you keep doing a chore simply because you can't stand looking at the mess, you will eventually 'own' that chore. It won't occur to your partner to say thank you since you're just 'doing your job'. When you recognise this you have the tools to fix it. My partner thought I loved picking up his clothes since I always picked them off the floor and put them away. He was genuinely surprised when I told him I was sick of doing it. My daughter is oblivious to the dishwasher; she thinks dishes move from the sink to the dishwasher to the cupboards overnight by something akin to the sorcerer's apprentice or osmosis as I put them away because I can't bear to see them stack up in the sink.

If you do more than your share of housework here are some solutions:

- Avoid repeatedly doing a chore that you don't want to get stuck 'owning'.
- Tell your partner and children when you think a chore should be done, instead of waiting for them to reach their own threshold.

If you usually do less than your fair share of the chores, try to:

- Do chores before they become necessary.
- Create a schedule for specific chores, and stick to it.

To increase your satisfaction and happiness, both partners should remember to express appreciation for the work the other one does, even if it's not important to you.

One of the most important things you can give your children is a happy, stable marriage. Although you should not fight in front of them, seeing parents disagree and make up is not damaging as long as you argue in a way that is constructive. When children see others disagree and resolve it, it allows them to go out into the world with the same skills and not to fear disagreements. One of the reasons teenagers can be so difficult is that they argue with their parents on every point. This can be exhausting. However, what helps is to remember that they are learning the debating and negotiating skills that they will need in adulthood and these skills are essential for their confidence. The only people they can practise on are their parents and they do need to practise a lot. My daughter is so challenging but I am glad she stands up to me and disagrees. The only way our children can assert themselves and confidently say no when pressured into drugs, sex, drinking etc is if they have had enough practice and freedom at home in saying no and being heard and respected for their opinion.

9. AVOIDING EXAGGERATIONS AND GENERALISATIONS

You may not be aware but most of us do this. We escalate the negative – you always, you never, you don't, you won't – when we talk about our loved ones' behaviour. Don't exaggerate with you CAN'T SEEM to, you are USELESS at (and don't do this to yourself either). Keep it about now.

We are also guilty of negative interpretations – you did that deliberately to hurt me, wind me up etc. When you always assume someone is deliberately acting against you, you are thinking the worst of them, which goes against their need to be accepted and not rejected.

10. DON'T MAKE YOUR RULES MORE IMPORTANT THAN YOUR RELATIONSHIP

We have relationship rules and each person in a relationship brings their own rules which the other partner often does not understand or even know about. For instance, if you believe that when someone insults you you must walk away and maintain your dignity, and you marry someone who believes you don't walk away in a fight, you are going to fight about your behaviour instead of the issue.

If your rule is to sleep on a fight/problem and your partner's is to stay up until it is resolved you are going to have major conflict and even more to fight about. If your rule is to never shout and your partner's is to get it off their chest you will end up fighting about that instead of the issue you were initially fighting over. If your rule is to be openly affectionate and your partner's is to only show affection in private, if your rule is to do everything together and your partner's is to have time alone, you are going to argue about that. You must discuss with your partner what their rules are and decide what is more important – your rules or your relationship. We do need relationship rules but they must be jointly decided. You must work together on important rules. When we are newly in love we are very yielding but this does not last.

We go to a job that has clear rules and boundaries but come home to rules we don't know, understand or agree to. You must work together and, at times, you must decide who is in charge. Couples need to write these out and even display them prominently.

Your soul mate may be nothing like you. Don't try to make your partner be like you; instead, celebrate the difference. Liking and respecting the other person is more enduring than being in love.

Meeting your partner's needs is the basis of a relationship. Couples with long-lasting relationships work to avoid the above.

How to Argue Constructively and Confidently

Arguing is okay as long as you argue on the subject.

The definition of a good relationship is how couples argue and, even more importantly, how they end the argument. Relationship experts can predict if a relationship will last just by observing how couples argue.

It is unrealistic to expect to never row and never disagree. You only have to be around a group of two-year-old children to witness fighting and disagreeing about ownership of toys or sibling jealousy.

In today's world with each partner having probably experienced a lot of independence prior to the marriage, and with many families now a mixture of children from previous relationships all living together, arguing will happen. The key is to argue productively.

Do you deal with the issue or move into verbally attacking and insulting each other and name calling? Not arguing is unrealistic; you just need to argue in a productive way that works for both of you.

Look at how you argue and learn to argue differently and effectively. If you are arguing about your partner's spending habits and digress into rowing about the fact that they are always late, don't do the laundry or forgot your birthday, you can't resolve the spending issue. To have healthy disagreements only argue about the issue/subject and don't veer from it. If you are arguing about the fact that your partner comes home too late from work each night, don't sidetrack on to a different issue such as how messy they are, how they spend too much money, they don't like your family, never put petrol in the car etc. Stay on the time they get home issue.

- Work towards resolving it. The whole point of arguing is to find solutions. You are not arguing to make someone else wrong or to make them feel bad or to point out how useless they are and how superior you are. You are arguing to resolve something so do it in a confident, productive, solution-orientated way as if you were at a business meeting, which means treating the other person with respect.

- Don't interrupt. You have two ears and one mouth for a reason – to listen more and talk less. When you respect the person enough not to interrupt you then have leverage and confidence to ask them to do the same, which means they will listen to you, so you don't need to keep repeating yourself. It's no longer necessary.
- Argue like an adult. Name calling is childish and also counter-productive. It does not help you to resolve anything and if you would not argue like this at work then don't do it at home. Character assassination does not have any benefits so don't fight dirty by insulting the other person. It just makes you look as if you have no negotiating skills and have to resort to name calling. If you want to grow in confidence see your arguments as negotiations and you will deal with them in a more effective way.
- Good communication skills are talking about you not the other person. Many arguers talk about the other person, who already knows what they do. Your partner knows what they did and you are giving them no insight into you and how you feel and inviting defensiveness when you say things like:
  'You do this, you said that, you went there, you forgot, you upset me.'

In order for your partner to understand you, you must express your feelings only, by saying things like:

I feel like this when	instead of	You make me feel
I get upset by	instead of	You do ———————
I get upset when	rather than	You upset me by
I was hurt about	rather than	You hurt me
I got angry over	not	You made me so angry

When you say I, you are explaining your emotions. When you say You, you are accusing the other person so explain, don't accuse, and you will become much more confident and successful at communicating and at resolving rows.

When you are responding to your partner don't say:

- I don't agree or You're wrong.

Instead say:

- I don't agree but I understand how you feel/why you feel that way.
- Just because I don't agree with you it doesn't mean I don't know how you feel.

Don't say:

- You are wrong.
- You're crazy.
- What are you on about?
- Have you got rocks for brains?

It is really important to say:

- 'I hear you, I get it that you feel this way.'
- 'I understand what you're saying/feeling even if I don't agree with it.'

We need to feel heard just as much as we need to feel understood. Feeling heard and understood increases our confidence.

Don't justify your behaviour or your partner's. Just say:

- 'I'm sorry you feel that way.'

For example, if your partner complains you are always home late, justifying is saying I have to work late to pay for everything. Instead say, 'I am sorry you feel like this and I understand why you do.'

- Learn to respond to conflict constructively and end the argument well so that you have no fear about further arguments. Don't go into punishing or refusing to speak to the other, refusing to hug or make up, but also don't feel you must have sex to make up if you don't want to. You can refuse sex without refusing affection. How you end a fight is a good indicator of whether you will stay together. Sometimes it is more important to be kind than it is to be right and it is always more important to do the right thing than it is to be right.
- Tenderness and kindness are not signs of weakness but of strength, inner confidence and resolution. People who apologise are confident, have high self-esteem and are very solution-orientated so be quick to apologise instead of slow.

The Confidence to Say 'No'

We get upset and frustrated in relationships when we hear no as it makes us feel powerless and not heard. A technique for superior relationships is to say no in a different way.

THE SANDWICH TECHNIQUE: HOW TO SAY NO

Your partner suggests sex. Don't say no. The sandwich works like this:

- I love having sex with you.
- I'm actually tired tonight.
- I would love to do it tomorrow and I am going to set aside some special time for us.

Your partner suggest going out:

- I would love to go to that new restaurant.
- I just don't feel that hungry tonight.
- Can we go on the weekend so I can really enjoy it?

Your partner suggests buying something you can't afford. Don't say:

- Are you kidding?
- We don't have the money.
- What a waste.

Say:

- I would love to own that.
- We can't afford it right now.
- Let's buy it next month/save up etc.

- The sandwich is the compliment.
- The filling is the refusal.
- Then a second compliment.

Couples I work with initially think the sandwich technique is cheesy but when put into practice it is amazingly effective and does not feel patronising.

If you are always saying no it creates a negative, controlling effect on the relationship.

Instead use words or expressions like:

- Later.
- Maybe next week.
- When we have paid off ——.
- We could put a deposit down and save up.
- Not now but definitely next month/year.

Your child asks you for something. Instead of saying no, you say:

- We can't buy that today but ——.
- When you have earned enough stars.
- At Christmas.
- When you are eight.
- Then we will get it.

If you want to paint your bedroom blue and your partner wants to paint it green, if you say to your partner 'I want it blue and I am not budging', you will reach stalemate very quickly. We often react very badly to criticism and ultimatums. A more effective way is to say, 'I would love this room to be blue' and to explain why and then leave them to think over their decision. We actually do love to please our partners but it is vital that we think it was our idea or that we wanted to do this or go along with it, not that we were bullied or forced into it. With all the couples I work with the happiest are those where the women often get their way but the men always feel it was their idea. I mentioned earlier that when my partner had cancer he found his own oncologist and I found the best oncologist in England for his type of cancer. When I asked him to see this person he said 'no', he was happy with the person he had found and he wanted to deal with this his way. I asked him if he would just talk to him on the phone, if he would consider a second opinion. I had to ask him quite casually as he was in a horrible situation and I did not want to pressure him in any way. When he made the call he found out that the oncologist I recommended had trained the oncologist he wanted to see. He got off the phone and said, 'I am going to see the teacher not the student.' This man probably saved his life and occasionally he says. 'I am so glad I found him.' He never mentions that it was me who found him and it does not matter. I don't need to bring it up because I understand his need to feel that he fixed his problem not me. Men don't like to feel that someone else fixed them as it makes them feel weaker, more beholden and vulnerable.

When a man's car develops problems and he tells a male colleague, that colleague will tell him, 'I know someone who can fix it', give him the details and the issue is sorted and finished. Women may get the same information but they then want to talk about how it feels to have a car break down and what it was like to be stranded on the roadside. This is hard for men who want to fix everything but not to talk about it, whereas women often want to talk about things but not fix them, which men don't understand. Women have to show them that they want to be listened to and heard without necessarily being given a solution. This is also empathy. I was telling one of my male patients to murmur, 'Oh, poor you' when his wife told him she had got three parking tickets in a week. She did not want him to say, 'Why don't you put more money in the meter or go by public transport?' She already knew that as she was an intelligent woman: she wanted sympathy and empathy. He told me later, 'It took me twenty years to learn to say, "Ohhhh, poor you" and it has changed my marriage. I only wish I had known it before.'

Listening to your partner will allow you to see that when we complain about our day we don't expect our partners to fix it by saying, 'Why don't you get a new job/End that friendship/Tell that person how you feel?' We want our partner to say, 'Oh, that's horrible for you.' Even saying nothing but 'Oohhh, sweetie' will get better results than saying:

- 'Well, you should have ———'
- 'Could have ———'
- 'Ought to have ———'
- 'Well, why didn't you ———?'
- 'What you needed to do was ———'
- Or, 'I would have ———'
- Or, 'I just don't understand why you put up with it.'

We fall in love with the opposite and it is vital to maintain that. Don't become too similar to your partner. Couples often begin to look and act alike. Wearing matching tracksuits and trainers means they are becoming too alike and losing themselves and the attraction they had for each other in the process. Your soulmate is not the person just like you. He or she may be nothing like you but you will learn and evolve in the relationship. Why would you want to be with someone who is just like you? What could you ever learn from that? Don't try to be like your partner and don't try to make them like you. Understand the difference without trying to change it. Opposites don't really get attracted to each other. It is the opposite polarity of male/female energy that attracts us to each other and that's why it's vital to stay male or female and vital to remain an individual in relationships while embracing the differences.

Looking into your partner's eyes is very bonding. Newly in love couples look into each other's eyes 70 per cent of the time. This is why newborns stare at their mothers and don't break the gaze as it is very bonding and creates oxytocin, a feel-good chemical. A technique of matching your partner's breathing and holding their gaze is a simple but highly effective way of feeling closer to your partner. The mechanical action of staring at your partner and not looking away brings on a bond of love as it is so intimate it also builds confidence. Lovers have the same body language as it creates harmony. When couples fight they deliberately put their bodies in opposing positions which accelerates the bad feelings. They fold their arms and stand with feet wide apart and turn their feet, hips, head and shoulders away from their partners; they often jab their fingers at their partners and scowl, their voice is hard and raised instead of soft and warm. This pose says, 'I want to be apart from you. I want to get as far away from you as possible.' In an argument if you make yourself come out of this pose and go into an open pose, you will be more in harmony with your partner on every level. Changing body language ends fights quickly and keeps couples in harmony.

Of course, you don't have to do all of this perfectly or remember all of it all the time, but if you do most of it most of the time you absolutely will have more confidence in yourself, in your communication skills and in your relationships. Just by ending destructive criticism and defensiveness and expressing your hurt you will feel so different and grow in confidence. It is worth printing out some of the things that are particularly relevant to you and sticking them on your fridge or your bathroom mirror so that you can always have access to them. I was working with a couple who were very unhappy and constantly argued and as I took them through the ten points one of them constantly rolled their eyes, sighed and grimaced (yes, that is contempt, scorn and mockery). However, at the next appointment that same person said, 'I have laminated your points and stuck them up in our kitchen and we are really getting on so well. It's working much better than I would have believed. Is it okay with you if I copy them and give them to some friends who are unhappy with their marriage as it's made such a difference to ours?'

STEP 8

Believing and Winning

In order to succeed in the business world you must have confidence in yourself, an inner confidence that radiates out to others. In the business world sales are all about confidence and making the customer believe in the product and in the person selling the product. Companies invest a lot of money in the psychology of selling which is very similar to sports psychology in that the most effective businessmen and women have to have a winning attitude and have to be able to come back from no and keep going. They cannot quit or give up when things get tough. I have worked with Olympic athletes and Premier League footballers as well as other successful sportsmen and women. I have also worked with top traders in the city and CEOs, and I use the same techniques with premier athletes that I use with premier business people, which is to instil in them an unshakeable confidence in their abilities and a drive to win, to make them feel that they can be and are the best. If you want to make it in the corporate world you must expect to win, and you must really want to win. That is what shows like *The Apprentice* are all about: looking for the person who has the winner's attitude, who will do whatever it takes, who is confident in themselves and in their abilities. It's also why on *Dragons' Den* no matter how good a product is, if the person making the pitch is not also good it won't get taken up.

Why Don't We Expect to Win Any More?

Many schools have taken away all elements of competition, believing it is bad for us, but children still love competing and as a nation we love the Olympics, the World Cup finals and, of course, the ever increasing amount of TV shows that have a big competitive element, voting off the losers and championing the winners. The drive to win to be the best in your field or amongst the very best, and the belief that you can win, must become a part of who you are in order to make it in the business world.

I'M A BELIEVER

'*Belief without talent can get you further than talent without belief*'

There are many studies to prove this with celebrities and pop stars who don't have outstanding talent but do have outstanding and phenomenal self-belief, and many people who started out in business with nothing more than a belief that they would make it and a determination to do whatever they had to do, who have made it. To make it you must always have belief in yourself. Ideally, this should be taught at school and in the schools where it is taught children have gone on to great success, but it is never too late to instil it in yourself.

Examples of people with ultimate self belief:

Richard Branson – Despite a poor academic record, Richard Branson began his first business venture at the age of sixteen when he set up a student magazine and then a music mail order business, before moving on to Virgin Records, then Virgin Atlantic Airlines, Virgin Trains, Virgin Mobile Phones and Virgin Media. He is now worth an estimated £1.6 billion.

Sir Alan Sugar – He began life in a council flat in the East End and left school at sixteen after a basic education. He now has an estimated fortune of £830 million from his technology and property portfolio.

Donald Trump – His business went into bankruptcy in 1991 but he always knew he would come back and persuaded his banks to continue to support him. His extraordinary confidence and self-belief influenced their belief in him and today he is worth $3 billion.

Arnold Schwarzenegger, Governor of California – Moved to America as a twenty-one-year-old bodybuilder. He spoke little English and had no money but was determined to become an actor and felt he was destined for great things. He said, 'I knew I was a winner back in the late sixties. I knew I was destined for great things. People will say that kind of thinking is totally immodest. I agree. Modesty is not a word that applies to me in anyway – I hope it never will.'

Muhammad Ali – He defeated almost every top heavyweight in his era. Ali was named Fighter of the Year more times than any other boxer. He was a masterful self-promoter, and his confidence and psychological tactics before, during and after fights became legendary. He is a shining example of ultimate self-belief. He said, 'It is a lack of faith that makes people afraid of meeting challenges, and I believed in myself. "I am the greatest," I said that before I even knew I was.'

Lance Armstrong – Tour de France champion who battled and beat brain, testicular and lung cancer after being given a less than 50 per cent chance of surviving. He not only regained his health but he won the Tour de France, calling it a victory over cancer. He has such a winner's attitude that he called the cancer 'the best thing that ever happened to me'. He also said, 'Pain is temporary. It may last a minute, or an hour, or a day, or a year, but eventually it will subside and something else will take its place. If I quit, however, it lasts forever.'

Martina Navratilova – She has always had a fantastic attitude and never minded being perceived as different as long as she was perceived as a winner. She said, 'Whoever said, "It's not whether you win or lose that counts" probably lost.'

Paula Radcliffe – Paula stated on record that she believes her single-mindedness, more than her physical prowess, gives her the competitive edge and makes her the fastest women in the world over twenty-six miles.

Stevie Wonder – He has not allowed being blind to hold him back in any way.

Simon Woodroffe OBE – He left school at sixteen with two O levels. He then went from being a roadie, to a stage designer, to the visionary founder of Yo! Sushi and Yo! Hotel, to a worldwide motivational speaker and panellist on *Dragons' Den*.

Believe and Receive

CHANGE YOUR BELIEFS INTO THOSE OF A WINNER

Beliefs affect everything we do and our identity beliefs – what we believe about ourselves – are the most powerful of all beliefs. The strongest force in all humans is that our body must act in a way that matches our thinking. If you feel not good enough, not confident enough or not up to your job you will act that way; if you feel uninteresting or less attractive than your colleagues you will give off that feeling to others. Identity beliefs affect everything – who you are, what you do, what you aspire to, even what you wear and what you eat. All beliefs can be changed if you introduce doubt. The minute we question a belief we no longer hold it to be true. That is why religion does not always allow us to question the priest, or rabbi, or imam as they do not necessarily want their beliefs questioned or changed. There are so many people who are hugely successful who were almost written off at school yet they did not accept the beliefs or opinions their teacher had of them.

THINK AND WIN

Change your Thoughts. What we think we are, we are. I use the story of the Vikings burning their boats to encourage athletes to perform without fear and to win. The Vikings burnt their boats so they had to win; they had no other option. There was no going back. We don't remember who got a silver or bronze medal, only the gold. Winning is everything. You must think like a winner to be a winner. It is essential to have a warrior attitude, to be a tiger not a pussycat. Arsène Wenger recently commented that Wigan play without fear. When I have worked with football players I also use the Viking analogy, that the only way to win is to go straight through their enemy, and it works. Diego Maradona would never think that being too small to head balls would disadvantage him as a footballer, and nor would Michael Owen. For years George Best did not believe his drinking affected his playing and for a long time, to the amazement of everyone, it didn't. He could see a goal from anywhere on the pitch. I use his belief system to have my clients see themselves as goal-scoring machines, unstoppable and goal-driven/orientated. You can benefit from this type of thinking whatever your career or profession. You can use these techniques to grow in confidence and to secure an interview and get the job, to win a client or contract, to get a promotion or to attract your ideal partner.

TALK THE WALK

Change your Language. Your brain uses the words you use to work out how you are feeling. Muhammad Ali never said, 'I am amongst the best or one of the best.' He said, 'I AM THE GREATEST. No one can beat me.' He fully believed it and so did his opponents. You have to think it, believe it, speak it and live it then you become it until It is no longer what you do, it's who you are.

GET A WINNER'S ATTITUDE

Change your Attitude as well as you Attire. When a businessman or woman puts on their work clothes they feel more professional because they feel they look the part. When women put on sexy clothes they feel sexier. The right clothing can change our attitude; so can the right thinking, which you are learning through this programme. Sports psychologists believe that everything can be taught to athletes except attitude, yet attitude is one of the greatest essentials in sport and business. The thing I love about my programme is that anyone can learn to have a winning attitude because hypnosis can install this in you, and since this book is written in a hypnotic style and the audio download is designed to change your attitude at a subconscious level, you can gain a confident attitude. Scouts looking for athletic talent and casting agents casting performers look for attitude first. They want those who have a warrior's mentality. Even on shows like *The X Factor* boot camp they won't put through talent that they feel can't cope with pressure. Head down is a loser's posture; they look for those who are upright and keep coming back, those who can take pain and keep going. You can learn to do this. Confucius said, '**Our greatest glory is not in never failing but in rising every time we fail**'. Businessmen who have been imprisoned, like Gerald Ronson, Jonathan Aitken and Jeffrey Archer, still see themselves as winners. Being in prison has not lessened their confidence; in fact, the latter two used their time in prison to write successful books and to campaign for improved prison facilities. Businessmen who have gone bankrupt will always come back as they have a template for success just as long as they don't see themselves as failures. When Donald Trump was more than a billion dollars in debt he still had a winner's attitude, he still lived in the style of a hugely successful, confident businessman and within a year he was out of debt and hundreds of millions of dollars in profit. Gerald Ratner of Ratners jewellers still had a winning attitude throughout his adversity. Kelly Holmes and Paula Radcliffe lost but came back to win as they refused to see themselves as losers. Ruth Badger did not see herself as a loser. When Christine Keeler and Mandy Rice-Davies were involved in a political scandal in the sixties Christine was broken by it whereas Mandy refused to be bowed and went on to have a happy, successful life. A few years ago Arsenal signed a sixteen-year-old for a record-breaking sum because he had spirit and a determined attitude that impressed them as much as his football skills. That footballer is Theo Walcott who, at seventeen years old, was selected for the England World Cup squad by Sven-Göran Eriksson.

Athletes who visualise can cause all their muscles to perform at a level to meet their visualisation. Very soon only athletes who can and do visualise will make it to the Olympics because they are so much better in every way than those who do not use this skill. If you are going for an interview or an assessment, if you are giving a speech or leading a meeting, visualise yourself as successful and you will be more successful.

The more you visualise the more you will believe your visualisation is possible. Very successful people visualise all the time and you have the visualisation scripts for increased confidence and success in Step 6 to help you as well as the scripts on the audio download. Changing the pictures we make and seeing ourselves doing what we want to do, and therefore not seeing the opposite of that, is a vital and relatively easy step. Everything we want, without exception, is because of how we think it will make us feel. What the mind sees it believes without question; your ability to visualise will have a powerful effect on you. As you visualise you will stimulate your mind and body into action. Remember: what you can hold in your mind with confidence you can achieve. At the top level, in addition to having the skill and talent required for success only those who can visualise peak performance, victory and unshakeable self-belief will come out ahead. Channelled properly, motivational thought processes and intense visualisation can be more powerful than pharmacology. You can use the hypnosis scripts in this book and on the audio download to constantly expand your potential. *Kazen* is a Japanese word that means constant and never-ending improvement. Your potential expands as you move towards it so you can never know what your potential is, and it's exciting to know you have as much unlimited potential as a top business person or athlete and that you can use it to increase your confidence and reap the benefits.

Change your habits. The way we feel is always linked to two things: the pictures we make in our head and the words we use. Changing our language and changing the pictures we make so that we see ourselves as confident winners and refer to ourselves as confident winners is a fast and permanent way to change, to make you more confident, more driven and more outstanding. If you think you can't do it, you can't do it, and if you think you can, you can. Adrenalin junkies link huge pleasure to extreme sports; they love triathlons, paragliding and free diving because they link pleasure to the high they get and they compete without fear. Successful business people love going to work; they love taking on new challenges and they go the extra mile. They do more than they have to do. The mark of a truly successful person is that they do more than is expected of them; they do what they have to do and then they do more. They give more. Maria Sharapova has an incredible mental attitude. She is impossible to read because she never loses determination and always has a winner's body language, even if she isn't winning. City traders are very like athletes and I have often taught traders the same techniques I teach athletes; it's all about having the confidence and the security to trade when it's right and to know when to stop. In life the only risk is not to take the risk.

Think of all the risks you have taken and how often it has worked for you. Asking someone out, asking for a job, asking for a pay rise – you can learn to be excited by risks rather than fearing them.

DON'T TAKE NO FOR AN ANSWER. PEOPLE WHO 'DON'T DO NO' CAN'T BE REJECTED

I am always impressed by people like Simon Weston, the Falklands War veteran who was burnt over 49 per cent of his body and horribly disfigured when his ship was bombed. He has always refused to see himself as a victim and even met and became friends with Carlos, the Argentinian pilot who bombed his ship. People like the opera singer Russell Watson, who went on to fight back to win against adversity, inspire us because they won't give up. There are so many people who have refused to take no for an answer and have eventually got what they wanted. Not accepting no is a measure of your faith in yourself and in your product and, of course, in the business world you are a product, so it's essential to see yourself as a fantastic, valuable, desirable product. The winner of 2007 *Britain's Got Talent*, Paul Potts, moved everyone with his ability to never give up on his goal of being an opera singer, and the 2008 winner, George Sampson, was rejected the previous year but came back against the odds, determined to win and, despite a medical condition that should hinder his dancing, he won. In *The X Factor* 2008 Alexandra Burke is a great example of not accepting no; she got through to boot camp in 2005 but did not make the live show and was devastated. However, she picked herself up and was confident enough to put herself through it again and she won. She is destined for a very different future because she overcame rejection and didn't accept 'no'. Very successful people don't take any notice of NO. They come back from rejection and use it as a learning experience. They do get rejected but they keep going and you can learn to do the same. Nigella Lawson lost her mother, her sister and her husband to cancer and yet she said, 'I refuse to be unhappy.' **Success is not never failing; success is how quickly you get back on track.** People don't realise the amount of time it takes to succeed so they give up. They accept no. People who succeed don't hear and won't hear no. We overestimate how much we can do in one year and underestimate how much we can do in five years. J. K. Rowling got several rejections for *Harry Potter*. She was also told there was no money in children's books but she didn't accept that and give in; she continued to submit her book, ignoring all the rejections, and she is now the biggest earning author ever. *The Sopranos* took five years to sell and during those five years of nos the writer was told it wouldn't succeed as it was too violent. It went on to be the most financially successful series on television and has been critiqued as amongst the best of all television dramas. *Gone with the Wind* was turned down fifty times. *Desperate Housewives* was turned down by HBO, CBS, NBC, Fox, Showtime and Lifetime. It took years to sell but is now the most popular show, in its demograph, worldwide. *The Shawshank Redemption* was initially a flop at cinemas but went on to have a huge word-of-mouth success. Erin Brockovich and Anne Anderson both took on huge American corporations and won against the odds because they would not accept no. Confident people never give up, they don't take no for an answer and they see any failure as an opportunity to learn something and move on. They never quit. This is the same confidence you were born with. The ability to not give up, to refuse, to quit or accept defeat, is how you learnt to feed yourself even though the first few attempts involved you getting food everywhere but your mouth – it's how you learnt to walk and talk, get dressed and do things for yourself. Confidence gets better and easier with practice. It also helps to remember that the first time you do anything that will be the hardest it ever is and then it gets easier each and every time. Hold that in mind as you overcome difficult tasks and minimise any adversity in doing something you have not done before.

The first time I used my sat nav I wanted to throw it across the motorway as it annoyed me so much that I could not work it properly. Now I can use it on autopilot. When I first began to give lectures I would only ever speak if I could have a podium to stand behind and hold on to as it masked the fact that I felt a little shaky and gave me somewhere to hide notes. Now I can give lectures without notes and without a podium as it has become second nature to me. Confidence is a natural talent we all have and, like any talent, if you practise you just get better and better. Many studies of the most successful athletes have concluded that it is practice that makes them better than the other athletes. The more you practise at something the better you become, the better you become the more you do it and the more you want to do it. We learn to speak at two and at twenty we are much more practised, at forty even more eloquent just because of all the practice. People who speak in public or speak professionally find the more they do it the easier it is and the more natural it all seems. Becoming confident at computers or cooking is so much to do with practice; if you do anything frequently it will become second nature, like living in another country makes you become confident about speaking the language simply because you get so much practice at it. That's how it is when we learn to drive or learn to operate a machine. First we go through the motions reminding ourselves what we have to do, then we do it automatically and eventually very easily and with confidence. By using this book you are to going to adopt and keep techniques that will enhance your happiness, self-esteem and confidence for good. Becoming naturally confident makes you happier. It makes you better at your job and it gives you empowerment in every area of your life.

Everything we see and use, from computers and telephones, machinery inventions, art and architecture to breaking world records, is because someone somewhere had confidence in their own ideas. They believed in themselves even when others laughed at them. In the early nineteenth century the authorities tried to stop steam trains from being developed as they believed that if a train travelled at over 30 mph it would cause pregnant women to miscarry and dry up the milk in cows in adjoining fields, and that human beings who exceeded that speed would be killed by the force of gravity. Luckily someone chose not to believe that and now we have bullet trains that travel at 186 mph, and in France the TGV set a record for travelling at 357 mph in April 2007.

When Roger Bannister ran the mile in under four minutes he instantly ended the belief that it was an impossible feat for a human to do. It was once believed that no one could possibly run a mile in under four minutes until Roger Bannister used visualisation skills to see himself running a mile in 239 seconds. Over and over again in his mind he saw himself crossing the finishing line in 239 seconds and he did – he broke a record and he broke a belief. That same year eight more people matched his achievement and the following year fifty-seven people ran a mile in under four minutes because he made it possible by changing a global belief. Very religious athletes, including Maradona, Pele and Muhammad Ali, believe God is with them, guiding them, and this belief makes them invincible. When Mark Spitz broke records and won seven gold medals at the 1972 Olympics he was a hero. Now his times would not be good enough to get him into an Olympic swimming team. Our potential expands as we move towards it and that means that none of us can ever know what our potential is, as our potential grows and develops as we reach towards it and it never goes back to where it was before. All we can know is that our potential is an unlimited and wonderful thing. One of the reasons we can be moved to tears by an amazing singing voice, an outstanding sporting achievement or a phenomenal actor on stage is because another human being, someone just like us, has done something amazing. It shows us that the potential of humans is unlimited. If you could travel back many hundreds of years in time with all the stuff you know you would be king of the tribe, the leader of the world, because what you know and can do has expanded from what your ancestors knew and could do. Believing in yourselves makes you keep going instead of quitting or giving up. When Richard Geer and Luther Vandross were called overnight sensations, they both said, 'That is the longest night of my life. I have been waiting for this for over twelve years.' Many successful people who appear to have had overnight success or easy success will tell you that their success involved lots of failures and rejections, but they kept going. Richard Branson apparently called his company Virgin because he was so naïve. When he started out selling music cassette tapes as a student, people would buy them, copy them then return them for a refund and he would give it to them. His mistakes helped shape him into the visionary and extraordinary success he is today.

One of life's great truths, and something that has helped me more than I can say, is to understand that '**What happens does not affect you; how you interpret it does**'. It is not an event that affects us but the meaning we attach to it and the interpretation we choose to give it.

Years ago I worked with a brilliant and very successful woman who told me that, when she was little, her parents had told her that they had tried to terminate the pregnancy but it had not worked and, when she survived it, they decided that she must be meant to be here. They were concerned she might find out from another relative so they made a point of telling her about it and told her how strong and special she was and how she must have a very special purpose in life and was here for a reason. Not long afterwards I worked with another client who had also survived a termination and she said, 'How could I ever amount to anything? My own parents didn't even want me. I was born with a strike against me.' The second person was less fortunate in that she did not have the positive parental reinforcement but they both had the same experience. One used it as a reason to succeed, the other as a reason to fail.

That's why I had you change your interpretation about rejection in Step 2. Once you can change the meaning of an event and make it positive, it can't hurt you. Once you can change the interpretation of an event so that you can say 'I learnt from that', it can't hold you back. When you can identify areas of your personality or your life that are preventing you from being the confident person you want to be, you can take action to change and this chapter is showing you how to be confident in your professional life.

To enjoy true confidence you must be able to like yourself. I know I keep repeating this point but it's because I really want you to get how crucial this is. Your punishment and reward in life are exactly the same. You go to bed every night and wake up every morning with yourself. This is wonderful when you like yourself and awful when you don't like who you are. You MUST like yourself and you MUST use this programme to ensure that you like yourself and that it's so easy and natural that other people like you, as you like them. This will free you from the desire to impress or to be fake. When you truly like yourself you don't need to impress anyone and you feel motivated and inspired, you have a good attitude and you will do the things you need to do to move forward. I want this to be who you are, not what you do, so to help this stick take a few minutes to do the exercise below.

Exercise 1

Write down every compliment you have ever been given or received. Think of and write out all the reasons why people like you.

Make the list as long as you can. Go right back to your childhood and schooldays to access every compliment and every reason people like you. Add in your own compliments to yourself and the reason you like you; this is very important. Remember: **the most important words you will ever hear are the words you say to yourself and believe.** Put the list somewhere you can see it and read it **every** day. By doing this you are massively boosting your self-esteem and self-worth, so don't skip this or do it in a half-hearted way. Give it 100 per cent and that's what you will get back: a 100 per cent improvement in your sense of self-worth, self-value, self-esteem and self-image.

The Rules of the Mind for Confidence

As you understand how your mind works you can fully influence your mind rather than being influenced by thoughts and behaviours that you don't want or need. Imagine if you bought the most up-to-date computer, or sat nav, or state-of-the-art mobile phone and it came with NO instructions: how would you use it? You might find that you could not use it at all or you could muddle through, but you would never get the best out of your machine, you could never use it to its full capacity and you would not get the excellent results that the machine was capable of giving you. This happens with humans. We come into this world with the most amazing computer-like brain that is capable of doing so much but there are no instructions that tell us how to get the best from ourselves, no manual that shows you how to programme yourself for success, and so we muddle through when we are capable of so much more.

We can buy an abundance of books telling us how to raise our children but they don't tell us how to show our children how to run their minds for success. You can find instructions on how to take charge of your body, weight and shape but there are far fewer books showing you how to run your mind. As you understand the rules of the mind you will have more understanding of yourself and how to programme yourself for success and lasting confidence.

1. Every thought or idea causes a physical reaction

Ideas that have a strong emotional content always reach the subconscious mind because it is the feeling mind. Once accepted, these ideas create the same reactions in the body again and again. To change negative reactions in the body it is important to change the ideas responsible for the reaction both consciously and subconsciously.

So if you have strong negative emotions linked to taking risks, like going for interviews or speaking in public, they will move into your subconscious mind and have a very real and negative effect on you. Whereas by changing fear to excitement you have strong positive emotions linked to interviews or public speaking and the effect your thoughts and emotions have on you is positive.

2. What is expected tends to be realised

The brain and nervous system respond only to pictures and images, regardless of whether the image is real or imagined. The mental image formed becomes the blueprint, and the subconscious mind uses every means at its disposal to carry out the picture. Worrying is a form of programming a picture of what we don't want, but the subconscious mind acts to fulfil the picture you are holding in your mind. Instead of worrying about doing something new or taking on more responsibility at work, decide to feel excited about it. Our performance is absolutely linked to our mental pictures and expectations. If we expect to fail, if we say, 'I just know I will forget what I need to say', 'I know I will blush', 'I am bound to mess it up' then we will. Instead of expecting to fail, expect to succeed fabulously. Expect to feel as confident and as sure of success as you did as a baby and these expectations will be realised.

3. Imagination is more powerful than knowledge when dealing with the mind

Reason is easily overruled by imagination. Violence wouldn't exist if logic were able to overrule the emotional reaction. We can all stand on a piece of wood on the floor but if that piece of wood became a window ledge high up, the imagination of falling off becomes more powerful than the knowledge that we can stand there if we have to. Any idea accompanied by a strong emotion such as fear, or anxiety is more powerful than any logical information meant to disprove it.

Your imagination and your ability to see yourself as confident and self-assured, to believe you can increase your self-esteem, is powerful and will give you the desired results. It can help you deal with bullying and aggression at work by giving you the confidence to calmly stand up to workplace bullies by applying the things you learnt in Step 3.

4. Each suggestion acted upon creates less opposition to successive suggestions

Once a suggestion has been accepted by the subconscious mind it becomes easier for additional suggestions to be accepted and acted upon. So if you agree that this book has already caused you to accept some new suggestions then you know that this alone is making it easier for your mind to accept further beneficial suggestions. That's why it's so important to do all the written exercises as they ensure that you let go of old beliefs and lock on to new ones. If you have missed any just go back and do them now.

5. An emotionally induced symptom tends to cause organic changes if persisted with long enough

It has been acknowledged by many doctors that more than 75 per cent of human ailments are functional rather than organic, meaning that the function of an organ or other body part has been disturbed by the reaction of the nervous system to negative ideas held in the subconscious mind. We cannot separate the mind from the body so if you dread change and constantly focus on any failures, mistakes and disappointments, then in time negative organic changes must occur. If you welcome and enjoy change and challenges, and expect to be liked and to like people and to like yourself, then positive, organic changes must occur.

6. When dealing with the subconscious mind and its functions, the greater the conscious effort, the less the subconscious response

Willpower is not the tool to use when bringing about change. Haven't we all tried to remember something, tried really hard, and yet haven't remembered it, and then, as we stop trying, the information we are looking for comes to mind? This is because the more conscious effort you make the less the subconscious responds. Trying to go to sleep doesn't work for an insomniac. If you wake up from a dream that has occurred in the subconscious mind then try to remember it consciously. It does not really work. It is easier to close your eyes and go back into a subconscious state to recall the dream. When you are making physical changes by using physical exercise it's true that the more effort you put in the more results you will get back. But when you are making inner changes, when you are changing your thoughts, beliefs and expectations, the opposite applies. You don't need to try; you just need to let your subconscious mind absorb these new ideas, accept them, have new expectations which will be met. When making mental changes effort is not truly necessary. What is necessary is the ability to get an image of how you plan to be and to hold that image in your mind, relax into the image and use language that matches the image, and keep rerunning the image so you are rehearsing it to such an extent that your brain thinks, 'I have been here before, I know how to do this, it is easy.' As you take on new beliefs about your innate confidence you will replace all the old negative ones but you must do it fully. You must programme your subconscious mind specifically. Form good images about your talents and abilities in your subconscious mind, which is the feeling mind and can remove, alter or amend old ideas and beliefs for good. The only work and effort involved is the written part of the exercises and these are very important. And, of course, there are things you don't have to *do* but to consciously *not do*, like criticising yourself. Again, this isn't work, it's just something to be aware of and to stop doing.

7. Once an idea has been accepted by the subconscious mind it remains until it is replaced by another idea

The companion rule to this is:

8. The longer the idea remains, the more opposition there is to replacing it with a new idea

Once an idea has been accepted it tends to remain. The longer it is held the more it tends to become a fixed habit of thinking. This is how habits of action are formed, both good and bad. First is the habit of thought and then the habit of action. We have habits of thinking as well as habits of action; however, the thought or idea always comes first. So if we want to change our actions we must begin by changing our thoughts.

We have many thought habits which are wrong but are still fixed in the mind. Some people believe that at certain times they must have a beta blocker to cope with speaking in meetings or a cigarette to calm them down. This is not necessarily true. The beta blocker they take could even be a placebo, but the idea is there and it is a fixed habit of thought.

There can be opposition to replacing it with a correct idea. These are fixed ideas not fleeting thoughts, but no matter how fixed the ideas are or how long they have been held they can absolutely be changed.

CONVICTIONS

Only use convictions for things that are beneficial to you. Become convinced that you can do it instead of convinced that you can't; become convinced that this book is working for you and convinced that the changes it is making in you are permanent.

OPINIONS

Opinions can easily be changed because they are often temporary, based on information. That's why it's so useful when someone says, 'You can't do that' or 'You should not, must not do that' that you just reply or say to yourself, 'According to whom? Who decided that and what did they know? Who said I shouldn't and where is it written that they are right?' Just because a parent said, 'Don't draw attention to yourself, don't make a fuss, don't have ideas above your station', that does not have to be and must not be your opinion. I have clients whose parents and grandparents would say things like, 'Don't show yourself up' because they wanted to be a performer, 'Don't ask for a discount, it's embarrassing', 'Don't work for yourself, you will have no job security.' If you were meant to be like your parents and grandparents there would be no point in you being here, and if we didn't challenge other people's beliefs, opinions and convictions life would never advance. All beliefs can be changed if you introduce doubt. The minute you begin to question something you no longer really believe it. After all, you believed in Father Christmas and the Tooth Fairy once and then you questioned it, doubted it and changed your belief. Now look at all your beliefs about your talents, your confidence, your sense of self-esteem and self-worth: are they opinions or are they convictions? You have all the information via this book to allow you to introduce doubt into any belief, conviction or opinion about yourself that is negative and has no benefit or useful purpose for you.

9. The Mind Cannot Hold Conflicting Beliefs

The mind also cannot hold conflicting thoughts. We can't be confident and anxious at the same time or happy and sad simultaneously. If you hold conflicting beliefs it sends the mind into a spin. It blocks the mind.

Making lots of jokes about failing, referring to yourself as a jerk or a loser does this. We cannot plan to succeed and then engage in joking about all our weak points because the beliefs are contradictory. They confuse the mind, which has to take literally everything we say as the truth.

I mentioned earlier that we are run by what we link pain and pleasure to. People who are successful in any area, i.e. relationships, health, career, have very clear definitions. If you want to be hugely successful but link pain to hard work or not having your weekends free, then you have mixed associations which you must change. If you want to become a fantastic salesman but can't talk to strangers, if you want to be a trader but are scared to take risks, you have conflicting beliefs.

Choosing our beliefs and changing beliefs that don't benefit us makes our life so much easier and humans are the only creatures able to do this. You cannot plan to increase your confidence and take more risks while dreading the process.

We first make our habits then our habits make us. People with addictions commonly give up the action but not the thought that runs it. Thought always comes first and it's vital in changing any behaviour to change the thought patterns that run it. What our mind sees it believes without question. Your mind has no capacity to reason; it believes whatever you tell it. One of the rules of the mind is that your body MUST act in a way that matches your thinking. Since thoughts always come first your mind influences your body and it can never be the other way round. A habit of action is run by a habit of thought. If your habit of action is putting things off or avoiding difficult tasks, and your habit of thought is 'It's too painful, too difficult, too risky, I'm too shy', you have to give up the habit of thought as well as the habit of action in order to achieve and sustain real confidence. An example of this is eating chocolate. Eating it is a habit of action but it's run by a habit of thought that says, 'This is something so good and it makes me feel better.' If you simply give up the habit of action but hold on to the habit of thought, you will always return to chocolate. The same thing happens if your habit of action is smoking and your habit of thought is 'Smoking relaxes me and helps me concentrate.' You can only succeed at changing the action habit if you also change the thought habit. People frequently put all their energy and attention into giving up the action while still believing the same thoughts, which is why they don't get lasting results. If you think you can't do it, you can't do it, and if you think you can, you can. Throughout this programme you are subtly changing your thought habits, so changing your action habits becomes a conclusion to this. Of course, thoughts don't start off as ingrained habits but once an idea has been accepted it tends to remain until it becomes a fixed habit of thinking. This is how all habits are formed. First comes the habit of thought then the habit of action. Babies don't blush because they don't have a habit of thought that says, 'I am embarrassed at being the centre of attention or being seen naked'; that then leads on to the habit of blushing and young children don't stutter because they don't have a habit of thought that says, 'I can't speak to strangers' that precedes the stuttering. The thought or idea always comes first. If you want to change your actions you must begin by changing your thoughts. When you begin to question something you no longer really believe it. I am amazed at how many of my patients tell me, 'I have always been insecure. I was born like this. I have never had any confidence. I've never been able to talk to people.'

Look at all your beliefs about what you can and can't do. You can introduce doubt into any belief, conviction or opinion you have that is negative about you. This is especially true if you have a belief that you cannot succeed. The difference between confident people and those who lack confidence can be narrowed down to their habits of thinking and their habits of action. Habits can be either good or bad. Confident and successful people only have good habits. The more empowering habits you have, the better your life will be. Simon Weston came back from the Falklands War horribly maimed. He did not allow himself to see himself as a victim and went on to marry a gorgeous woman and have children because of his convictions that the person inside was still the same and because he refused to be a victim. Sir David Murray, the chairman of Glasgow Rangers Football Club, lost both his legs in a car crash and his wife to cancer but never sees himself as a victim.

Work through the following quick exercise to see just how powerful your thoughts are.

Exercise 2

As you read through these next few lines just imagine that you are standing in your kitchen and you are holding a lemon that you have just taken from the fridge. It feels cold in your hand. Look at the outside of it, the yellow waxy skin that comes to a small green point at both ends. Squeeze

---

it a little and feel its firmness and its weight. Now imagine raising the lemon to your nose and smelling that unique fresh lemon smell. Now imagine cutting the lemon in half and inhale it. The smell is stronger. Now imagine biting deeply into the lemon and letting the juice swirl around in your mouth. Taste the sharpness, the fresh citrus flavour. At this point if you have used your imagination well, your mouth will be watering.

Consider the implications of this. Words, mere words, affected your salivary glands. The words did not even reflect reality, but something you imagined. When you read those words about the lemon you were telling your brain you had a lemon. Although you did not mean it your brain took it seriously and said to your salivary glands, 'She/he is biting a lemon, hurry, wash it away.' Your glands obeyed.

If something as simple as imagining you were eating a lemon can cause your body to react physically then something as simple as imagining you are confident, self-assured and that you like yourself can and will cause your body to react physically.

Words do not just reflect reality; they can create reality – like the flow of saliva you just caused by doing the exercise. The subconscious mind is no subtle interpreter of your intentions; it receives information and it stores it, it believes without question everything you tell it since its job is not to question but to act immediately on your instructions, which to your subconscious mind are commands. Tell your subconscious mind something like 'I am eating a lemon' and it goes to work. That experiment was neutral, so physically no good or harm can come from it, but good as well as harm can come from many of the words we use.

If you are on an aeroplane waiting to fly abroad you may be filling your mind with images of the beaches or bars you are going to visit, the weather you are going to enjoy, and you will respond to those images. The person next to you may be filling their mind with images of fear; they may believe that some of the passengers look like terrorists and, as they focus on the fact that the plane may crash, they will respond to those images by becoming agitated and nervous. So two people on the same flight are responding differently because of the words and images they are creating.

The way we feel at any given time is due to:

- The pictures we make in our head.
- The words we say to ourselves.

The good news is that we can change those words and pictures at any time and we can learn to make them more positive all the time.

How to make Confident Affirmations Work for You

An affirmation is simply a short statement you repeat to yourself over and over for a few minutes daily, something like:

- 'I have ultimate confidence' or
- 'I have regained the huge amount of self-esteem I was born with'
- 'I like myself and I believe in myself'

You repeat it over and over out loud to yourself to allow your subconscious mind to accept it, but this will not always happen instantly because we often pick an affirmation that conflicts with some beliefs we may have. One of the reasons we are covering affirmations in this step is because by now you will have changed some beliefs and will be open to the idea of changing more. Many people give up with affirmations because their mind may seem to have so many objections to them; they don't really believe what they are saying or understand that there is a system for having the mind accept and believe affirmations, so they find the process frustrating and abandon it.

I have found that the best way to overcome this is to write out each affirmation as a statement and then just notice any objections that come to mind. Next, write out each objection your mind may come up with, keep on writing out the affirmation and writing out any objections or thoughts that come to mind directly underneath the affirmations in a notebook. It is important not to spend time attempting to analyse the objection. Just write them out and keep going.

It is worth writing out each affirmation and the consequent objection until you have exhausted and run out of all your objections. As you then review the response and the objections written out in your notebook you will notice quite a distinct pattern emerging because the more you keep writing out the affirmation the less objections your mind will come up with. Eventually you will run out of objections and move into acceptance that YOU ARE CONFIDENT, WITH HIGH SELF-ESTEEM.

Here is an example: you decide to say out loud each day as your affirmation I HAVE ULTIMATE CONFIDENCE.

Your mind may immediately come up with some objections, especially if you have been conditioned by the beliefs of others. These may be something like:

- You will be arrogant if you think like that.
- My friends won't like me if I have so much confidence.
- I will be a fake if I do that.
- How can anyone change that easily?
- Everyone will laugh at me if I do this.
- This is all rubbish.
- I don't believe in this.

Just keep going until you run out of objections, then you can add:

- Actually, I do believe in this.
- There are examples of people turning their lives around.
- If other people can do it so can I.
- Okay, it's true. I can and will have ultimate confidence.

As you continue to write out each affirmation and to say it out loud, your objections will become weaker and weaker, you will pay them less and less attention and your belief in your affirmation will become stronger. Eventually your mind will run out of objections and will then fully accept the affirmation. The good news is that since you are the one coming up with all the objections you can end the objections, stop letting them in and stop letting them effect your confidence.

Get into the habit of repeating your affirmations daily. Make sure you say them out loud. It doesn't matter if you feel silly; most people do initially. Just become aware of how you feel and the thoughts and feelings coming up as you repeat each affirmation.

It also helps to repeat your affirmations at night just before you go to sleep and again in the morning, just after waking, when your subconscious is most receptive. It is a very good idea to write out your affirmations and to stick them up on a mirror, or on the fridge door, to put them up as your screen saver or on your desk and anywhere else that suits you and causes you to remind yourself of them regularly and frequently.

By doing this you will be able to make your life and yourself and your ability to increase your self-esteem, self-confidence and self-image an ongoing, breathing affirmation. You will develop more and more potential through the use of your affirmations because the words and images you repeat over and over to yourself become the blueprint for who you become. Positive affirmations go into the subconscious and eventually replace negative thoughts. The subconscious responds the most to clear, authoritative commands. The more clear, precise and straightforward they are the more rapidly the mind accepts them and goes to work on them.

Affirmations can also build self-esteem, make you optimistic and diminish negative self-talk.

Now that you have your new confidence and it's here to stay, there are so many ways you can use it and benefit. You can have the confident manner to negotiate a discount or an upgrade with hotels, phones, car hire or shops. The most important thing to remember when you are asking for a discount is to never ask a question that can be answered with no, i.e.:

- 'Can I have discount?'
- 'No, we are not allowed.'
- 'Can you reduce this/mark it down/take off 10 per cent?'
- 'No, that's not possible.'

Instead, ask a question that is a statement:

- 'What is the very best price you will give me on this item?'
- 'What is the maximum you can take off the price for me?'
- 'How much are you going to reduce this by?'
- 'I understand you can reduce this for me by 10 per cent'
- 'What extras will you include in the price?'
- 'What will you give me as an incentive to buy it from you; free delivery accessories etc?'

When you ask, 'What is the best price you will sell this to me for' you are already making a statement that they will lower the price for you and now you are negotiating how much. You can do this in major stores, electrical chains, anywhere at all. I negotiated a great discount on a coat I wanted in Harrods. You must always be polite and give off an air that you expect a discount and are fully prepared to walk away and take your custom elsewhere if you don't get one. Even stores that say they have a no-discount policy will offer you other things like accessories, or a free warranty, or free delivery in order to make a sale.

It's the same when you are complaining about a service or returning goods. It is most effective if you can state in a calm, confident and firm yet pleasant voice, 'I am very unhappy with this service and I expect a full refund or a full exchange.' Don't ever ask them what they are going to do about it; you must tell them what you expect so that they can meet your expectations. Always go straight to the top and begin with the manager so that you don't have to repeat yourself with an assortment of employees. Before you return any goods or complain about service, it is worth reading the Sale of Goods Act as, once you know what you are talking about, service industries will treat you with respect and consideration. Those words 'Actually, under the Sale of Goods Act you are legally bound to do something about it' always work. For instance, your mobile phone or computer doesn't work and the shop tells you to take it up with the manufacturer. You simply reply, 'I bought this item from you so under the Sale of Goods Act my contract is with you and therefore I expect you to do something about it and you can take it up with the manufacturer on my behalf.' With insurance companies you must ignore their instinct to reject your claim and threaten to report them to the insurance ombudsman. My daughter's phone was stolen from her in a restaurant by a gang of hoodies and the insurance company told me that she wasn't covered out of the home as it did not involve violence or threat. I wrote back to them and asked them what they thought a gang of hoodies did involve and told them that, unless they reconsidered my claim and replaced the phone, I would report them to the insurance ombudsman. They sent me another phone within three days. You will find an ombudsman for most service industries and their job is to help you, so don't take no for an answer if you know you are in the right.

What's the Difference Between You and an Achiever?

Achievers break all the rules. They don't take no for an answer. The things that make an achiever can be summed up by only three things. Achievers:

- Believe they are unique.
- Break every rule.
- Don't take no for an answer.

You can take on any of these attributes. Achievers are no happier than you and I unless they really like themselves. People who want to succeed, to make it or to be famous really want to feel special. We all want to feel special to someone and celebrities want to feel special to everyone. They have often never felt special before and believe that fame and celebrity will make this possible for them. It is fleeting, though, as fame can be very short-lived, so the feeling of being special does not last and the competition around, with so many others who all think they are special, can cause the feeling of not being special to resurface. The people who seek fame in order to feel special don't confront the childhood issues that caused them to feel so unworthy, and so even if they achieve worldwide fame they still feel unworthy deep inside.

The common denominator of every emotional problem is a feeling or a belief that we are unlovable; many people who feel unlovable or unworthy believe that being famous will cure and solve the problem. People want to become famous to feel special because they didn't feel special in their childhood. They crave and have a burning desire to be seen as special, to be treated as special and will do almost anything to get it so they have huge motivation and drive for fame. But it doesn't work because even when they have a huge fan base that appears to love, even worship, them they feel the love is not real. The fans love the star's looks, talent, body or lifestyle but the star feels that if they really knew them they would be disappointed, so the feeling of being unlovable is still there and still unresolved.

Marilyn Monroe, Princess Diana, Kurt Cobain and Paula Yates showed classic signs of feeling unlovable. A celebrity's huge fan base does not make them feel lovable. They are special to their fans but not to themselves and they have nowhere to go to get that feeling. They have the fame that they thought would make everything better; when it is not enough, and can even make things worse, there is nothing to aspire to so the celebrity may turn to drink, or drugs, or unsuitable relationships, or another form of destructive behaviour. Carrie Fisher and Jason Donovan both said that when they were at the top of their careers there was nowhere to go but down, so they accelerated the down by getting into destructive behaviour – drink, drugs etc. Britney Spears, All Saints and The Spice Girls all began at the very top; when your career has peaked in your early twenties it is especially hard to know how to follow that for the rest of your life.

We can look around and see who is being treated as special. Models, top athletes, politicians, actors and showbiz celebrities: politics and sport require talent. Models need beauty but showbiz attracts people who are not the most gifted and celebrities can get by with very little talent. A top surgeon cannot get a table at the best restaurant in town. A celebrity can. A celebrity doesn't have to pay for things; they get preferential treatment constantly. Celebrities crave fame to solve their problems, then want to be anonymous again when the fame becomes overwhelming and the lack of privacy just creates a new set of problems.

NEEDING TO BE SOMEONE

Having an average and fulfilling life seems just not good enough any more. Becoming a 'somebody' is what so many people strive for these days. But why? Are children born wanting to be celebrities? No: they just want to be loved and cared for. Their desire to be famous is due to the lack of love and attention given to them by their parents. Both parents working full time, combined with the lack of parenting skills, can lead to this phenomenon; those who are neglected and ignored look around to see what they can do about this situation. They soon discover that people are not treated equally in this world. They discover that some people are seen as better, more special and are given lots of love and approval, while others are not. Through news, advertising and television they notice that famous people are considered different by the public and are treated better than the rest of us. Wanting to become one of these people is now their mission to attaining added attention and therefore more love. Now they have found something they can definitely go after and, if the fame seeker finds some sort of notoriety, the media wants to know all about them. It leads the fame seeker to think; *now I must be special!* It also fills their need to be loved and wanted. But this is a false belief, because when the fame seeker finds fame they are surprised to discover that they are just as unhappy and lonely as they were before, but now more people know about it. This can also lead to 'the self-destructiveness of talent', when many successful people debase their talent because they feel they did not earn it or work hard enough for it. The drive to be somebody, to be famous, or to be an achiever can be brought about by an inner feeling of being unlovable that fame, success and achievement don't cure. The cure is to know that you are lovable, that you are enough and that you don't have to prove it to anyone but yourself and by this stage of the book and by frequently playing your audio download you will do just that.

STEP 9

Depression and Anxiety

- You, only better
- Finding your place
- Meeting your needs

I talked in Step 2 about our need to avoid rejection and in Step 4 about not feeling enough. When our needs are not met and we don't feel enough, it can lead to depression and a feeling of worthlessness and helplessness that seems insurmountable. However, depression can be overcome. Having worked with many clients, from the depressed to the suicidal, I have found that depressed people usually feel helpless and hopeless, useless, worthless and empty: they have almost no self-esteem. They often feel that they don't deserve help and believe that they are a burden on others and will never get better. They go far beyond the feeling of not being enough and feel that they are not worthy of or deserving enough of treatment or help and they can't see a solution. Because depressed people don't feel worth it, they have no motivation to take care of themselves with exercise or vitamins and the right food and instead usually don't eat correctly as they can't see the point of looking after themselves. They can often be resistant to seeking help, feeling they don't deserve to waste the time of those who could help them, and since they believe they can't be helped it all seems pointless. Depressed people only believe their own opinions and won't let in the opinion of others; they are a very good example of the fact that we only take in information that we choose to believe.

I have included in this chapter some case histories that you might relate to, as seeing how other people got better helps us all. When you understand what is really going on within you, that in turn can free you to get back your innate confidence and self-esteem as you will begin to recognise that it is not true that 'something is wrong with you and that you just can't help it and are destined to be like this for ever'; instead, you may find that it's incredibly empowering to identify the things that have been holding you back. Although the old thinking is that depression may be because of a chemical imbalance in the brain, recent studies (at the UCLA School of Medicine, using pet scans) show that changing negative behaviours can change brain chemistry. Many breakthroughs in neuroscience have shown that our brain continues to grow and develop throughout our lives. This means we can train our minds to be happy, to think positively, to reduce negative feelings and to choose how to feel and react to events that are going on in our lives. Negative behaviours and negative feelings come about because of negative thinking. I mentioned earlier that the mind cannot hold conflicting thoughts. When you are thinking negative thoughts you can't feel positive or happy, and when you are thinking happy, positive thoughts you can't feel negative. Many studies, including those of the eminent psychiatrist Dr David Burns, author of *Feeling Good*, show that the immediate cause of depression is harsh, hurtful, over-exaggerated critical statements that we put ourselves down with and beat ourselves up with on a regular basis, making us feel even more worthless and hopeless until it becomes a vicious circle. **Depression does not make you negative – being negative and critical about yourself on a regular basis makes you depressed.** It is our thoughts that can make us depressed, not the weather, the job, our financial situation, our looks or other people's behaviour (there are plenty of millionaires living in glorious sunshine who are depressed and numerous hugely talented, beautiful looking people who are also depressed). It is not even lack of love that causes depression. Many depressed people are much loved although they don't feel at all lovable. They just feel that they are a burden. Experts believe that we can give ourselves literally thousands of negative messages a day: that's enough to make anyone depressed.

When you are depressed you feel bad because you are thinking bad thoughts. You filter out all the good and focus on all the negative until, eventually, you only see, feel, think and talk about what is so bad about YOU, which in turns makes you feel worse. This is not conscious behaviour. No one wakes up with the desire to make themselves feel as bad as possible by focusing on everything bad. It is unconscious behaviour but because you aren't aware of this you just think everything about you is negative because you feel so bad, rather than realising that you feel so bad because you focus on the negative. I mentioned earlier that whatever you focus on you get more of and that the universe will support whatever you choose to believe, whether it is right or wrong, good or bad, helpful or unhelpful, uplifting or depressing. I also mentioned that the only difference between happy and unhappy people or depressed and undepressed people is their habits of thought and their habits of action. Negative thinking is a bad habit and, like all bad habits, this is one you must end and quit; give it up; replace it with something better. If you have been criticising and diminishing yourself for years, you will need to repeat your new habits until they lock in, and you know how to do that now because of the sections in this book on habits in Step 1 and Step 8. Your negative habits are not conscious but by making a conscious effort to change them you can succeed at overcoming depression. This may sound way too simplistic, and is not meant in any way to trivialise how paralysing depression feels for those in the grip of it. However, once you can accept that depression is because of the way you see yourself and the way you talk about and diminish yourself, you will be able to silence your inner critic for good. Step 3 has already shown you how to do this but I recommend you read that section again when you have finished this chapter.

When we feel depressed we feel different. We feel that no one can understand us or relate to us and we can't relate to them, so we feel isolated and we can't feel that sense of connection that is essential to our happiness. Connection is an essential need, as is feeling significant; we also need diversity and certainty. Diversity means we need things to not always be the same; we need good change and certainty is a feeling that everything will be all right. Of course, as a child we depend on our parents to meet these needs and if they don't we can go through life feeling unable to get our needs met, which in turn causes depression. We have other needs for growth and contribution along with, of course, our strongest need to be accepted and not rejected, and in Step 10 and at the end of the book you will find very effective ways to meet all your needs.

Depression has a paralysing effect. It stops motivation and saps and eats away at willpower, replacing it with apathy, inertia and more depression. Depression affects your relationship with yourself and your relationships with others because it makes you want to shut yourself away from people. Clearly while you are in this state none of your essential needs can be met and when these needs aren't met this vicious circle leads to further and more severe depression. When you are depressed you don't feel like doing anything so you don't do anything, and this lack of action makes you more depressed and more isolated. Almost all countries, regimes and institutions have used banishment, isolation, solitary confinement, marooning, being cast out and being sent to Coventry as the worst type of punishment. Condemning someone to isolation is guaranteed to bring on depression. We would protest if that happens to animals in the zoo. Yet depressed people do that to themselves; because they feel so worthless their negative conditioning tells them that they can't cope with the pressure of seeing others and feeling they have to smile or be cheerful in their presence, so they prefer to be alone, and being alone and cut off from people and activities only serves to increase the depression. Psychologists have found that increasing the number of social contacts a sad person has makes them happier. The *Journal of Psychological Science* found that happy people spent the least time alone and the most time socialising with others.

CHANGE YOUR BEHAVIOUR AS WELL AS YOUR BELIEFS AND THOUGHTS

Changing your thinking changes your feelings but with depression it is essential that you also do some activities, because doing something that requires activity, no matter how small, can also change the depression. The way you act and the actions you take will change the way you feel. To cure yourself you must do the opposite of depressed behaviour. Feelings follow behaviour, therefore you must do what you don't want to do to end depression. Don't wait until you feel better to take some action. Do it now. Remember that I told you earlier you don't have to be motivated to do it; when you do it you become motivated. Don't wait for motivation or an improvement in mood before you take action; take action and you will become more motivated and get an improvement in mood.

You Only Better

These are some of the things you must do to diminish depression:

- Exercise, even thought you don't want to. Exercise releases endorphins which promote wellbeing and benefit our physical and mental health. You don't have to go the gym every day; even going for a walk helps, taking up yoga is particularly helpful and if you can take yourself to the gym or for a run, no matter how brief, you will feel better. Another effective cure for depression is movement through dance or tai chi. Exercise has a positive effect on brain cells.
- Touch is very important in healing depression. If you are depressed the last thing you feel like is sex; however, touch releases endorphins and the hormone oxytocin, so don't become touch-deprived: stroke pets, hug friends and family, resume sex with your partner or have a massage. It is so important to do the opposite of what you feel like doing and it will help you feel significantly better.
- Diet can play a huge part in curing depression; avoiding caffeine and sugar are particularly important as caffeine and sugar feed anxiety. Make sure you eat well and regularly, even if you have no appetite. Avoid all sweeteners as they can affect the brain and our moods in a very negative way. It is essential for our mental health that we eat good fats on a regular basis. Many people only eat bad fats like trans fats or saturated fats or try to avoid fat altogether. Make sure your diet has plenty of nuts and seeds, good oils like avocado and olives and oily fish or fish oil supplements. Getting the rights fats in your diet is vital for good mental health. Essential oils are just that: <u>essential</u> for your mental well-being, so eat them daily.
- Uplifting music can have a very powerful effect on our moods.
- Look into the future and know that it won't last, that it is not permanent, even though that does not seem possible at the time. Talk to other people who have felt so low and felt there was no way out only to have found that they fully recovered.

- When you regularly take on the physiology of a happy person, even though you may have to force yourself to do it, you will begin to feel happier. The more you practise being confident and happy the more it will become your natural and automatic state. At Bellevue Psychiatric Hospital in America doctors did an experiment in which they had the most depressed patients take on the physiology of someone who was happy, which simply required them to smile many times a day – the really big smiles that make your face crinkle – and to take on the body language of someone who was confident so that they stood upright rather than stooping or slouching. The results were astounding and proved that practising being happy and confident makes you more happy and confident. When you smile you make serotonin, which is known as the happy hormone.
- Vitamin B6 also increases serotonin. A lack of vitamin B3 can cause depression, while a lack of vitamin B6 can cause depression, inertia, insomnia and irritability. Lack of vitamin D, which is made in the skin by sunlight, is also linked to depression. Vitamin D levels can be increased by taking fish oils. B12 deficiency and low levels of Omega 3 can be an underlying factor in depression, so make sure you eat oily fish two or three times a week and take B6, B3 and B12 and Omega 3 supplements every day.
- Make sure you get outside for a while every day as daylight and sunlight increase serotonin. Many night workers and shift workers become depressed because of the lack of natural light. There are more examples of how to naturally increase your serotonin levels in Step 10.
- Laughter is an important antidote to depression. Many studies have shown that if you consistently watch funny films you make different chemicals from the ones you make when you feel depressed. Laughter releases endorphins and decreases stress hormones in the

bloodstream and has a positive effect on our bodies, which is why in his book *Anatomy of an Illness* Norman Cousins detailed how he rented funny films when he was very ill with cancer and watched them frequently, crediting the laughter therapy as playing an essential part in his recovery. You can boost your immune system and make feel-good hormones just by changing the way you think. At the Rainbow Children's Hospital in Cleveland, Ohio, an experiment was done whereby children watched a puppet show of a virus puppet fighting a policeman puppet who defeated the virus. After watching the puppet show the children closed their eyes and imagined lots of policeman puppets in their own bodies fighting their own viruses. Then saliva samples were taken that showed that the children's immune systems had reacted as if they really were fighting an infection and had made proteins to defeat the infection.

- Do what you love to do. Evidence has shown that when people don't follow their inner yearnings or do what they love, when they don't take up the career that they have a calling for or a deep need to be involved in, this can create depression, sadness, apathy and illness. So much depression is down to people not doing what they want to with their lives and suffering because of it. I worked with a client who was deeply depressed and had been for years because she had always wanted to be a lawyer but could never afford to attend law school and when she took early retirement she felt she had wasted her whole life. She could not get past the fact that she had missed out on working in law. Eventually we decided that she could still do something about it and after volunteering in a legal aid centre she did some training and became a magistrate, which does not require any legal qualifications. So finally she was working in a court doing what she loved and loving what she did and she was free of depression.

Another of my clients had always wanted to be a doctor but this was not possible for her as she did not have the funding or the education to go to medical school. She worked in a series of menial jobs and raised a family and at age fifty-five became depressed as her children had left home and her job was unrewarding. She began to comfort eat because she was alone and unfulfilled which made her more depressed and lethargic. When I worked with her it became clear that the depression was because she had never done what she really wanted to. Using the methods in Step 3 she began to ask herself how she could resolve this and what she could do about it. Her answer was to train to become an aroma therapist. She went on to work in a hospital and a hospice and found peace, contentment and tremendous job satisfaction because she was finally doing what she loved: working in a hospital and helping people in a hands-on way.

If you have always wanted to be on the stage, you can go to amateur dramatics or you can work backstage in the theatre. Another of my clients had always wanted to be a vet but failed his veterinary exams and was asked to leave veterinary school. He felt it was too demeaning for him to become a dog-walker or work at an animal shelter, but since he only wanted to work with animals he felt lost. His depression had closed in on him so he did not see that there were other options – it was not just black or white – eventually he trained to become an animal behaviour therapist and opened his own practice. He also worked on film sets, training animals for commercials and television work. He had a wonderful life that he enjoyed even more than if he had become a vet.

If you are depressed because you have not followed your heart's desire it is never too late to do something about it, and even if you can't make it your career you can still make it a hobby. One of my clients had never had children and was full of regret and deep sadness but eventually she decided to sponsor two children in Africa who she visited and wrote to regularly. While this was not the same as having her own child, it did help her and made her feel that she had children in her life and that she was making a difference to them and to herself. Don't live a life full of regrets about what you did not do, instead do something about it.

- Therapy with the right therapist is incredibly helpful. Evidence shows that effective talking therapy reduces over-activity in the part of the brain linked to anxiety.
- Medication has its place but it is not going to cure the thought process that may have caused the depression. To change depression you must change your thinking as well as your actions.
- To cure depression you must look at what role, function and purpose the depression is playing in your life. Is it allowing you to opt out? Does it free you from pressure or obligations? You may find some of the following case histories resonate with you and, if so, you can use them as a template for your own recovery.

Finding Your Place

When we don't feel certain that we belong to the group, which is our family or the people who are raising us, there are only four ways we can behave and each way is designed to reassure us that we belong and to make us feel secure within the group.

The first and statistically highest way we try to reassure ourselves that we belong is to become sick, to get ill, so that the group look after us, which then convinces us that we must belong after all or they would not go to so much trouble. Many of life's adult hypochondriacs and depressives get all their needs met through being ill as they get touch, attention, warmth, concern and caring and only feel important and significant when they are ill. However, because our need to be connected and significant is then met solely from being ill we don't feel loved for ourselves, which can in turn lead to more severe depression.

Case Study 1

I worked with a man in his mid-forties who seemed to have everything going for him except that he was plagued by a horrible depression, which would descend on him every Sunday afternoon and last for three to four days. It was what he called his black dog of doom and gloom in that it descended over him like a fog; he could not free himself from it and it was ruining his life. He could not enjoy weekends as he always expected it to arrive like clockwork on Sundays, and it did, and he could not enjoy the working week as it left him drained and unhappy. As he began to describe his symptoms to me I realised that something must be triggering his low feelings, so we talked about what Sunday afternoons meant and in hypnosis he went straight back to the cause. When he was nine he was sent to weekly boarding school and hated it. On his second weekend at home he asked his parents not to send him back; they refused and he became hysterical and ran off to stand in the river at the end of the garden so they could not get to him to send him back to school. Eventually they got him out and called over the local doctor who gave him some kind of mild sedative. Then they drove him back to school asleep and carried him into his dorm where he woke up the next day. This pattern seemed to continue. He would get upset and his parents would then put a sedative in his lunch and he would be returned to school in a dazed state and put to bed. He began to dread the whole Sunday afternoon ritual and long after his schooldays were over he still hated Sunday afternoons. He understandably had a lot of resentment towards his parents because of their actions, and this increased the depression, but he began to understand that, while his parents were absolutely wrong to do what they did, their intention may not have been bad, only their actions. Maybe they cared about him so much and could not stand to see him upset, which is why they gave him medication. The important thing was to change his interpretation of this event so that he was no longer full of resentment and bitterness, and to change the feeling that he did not fit in or have a place anywhere because he felt misunderstood and unhappy at home and at school. The belief that he did not fit in or belong in any place, and the feeling of never being understood and being insignificant, fuelled the depression and when these elements were removed the depression ended and he became confident and happy.

Case Study 2

Another of my clients, Suzie, had eczema on her face and arms and was so conscious of it that she became reclusive and depressed as the eczema affected her confidence and her self-image. Suzie recalled that as a child she got more attention than the other younger children as her mother would keep her off school so that she could be taken to various specialists. At night her parents would spend hours applying creams and bandages. It was the only time she felt more important than her baby brother and sister. Suzie did not like being the eldest and having to be responsible and look after the younger children; she felt she had no identity except as an extra carer and she wanted to be the baby, not to have to help look after it. By getting ill she had re-created her first few years when it was just her and her parents and by having the creams and bandages applied she was taking priority over the younger children and was allowed to feel like a baby and to feel like the most important child, being pampered and looked after. When she realised the link between the manifestation of the eczema and the fact that she no longer needed the attention it got her, because she no longer needed or wanted to be her parent's baby, it began to clear up, until it completely disappeared, along with the depression and the reclusiveness.

We don't all take on the role of being ill in order to feel that we belong. The second most effective way to ensure that we belong and are connected and secure within the group is to become a carer, to look after everyone in order that we make ourselves indispensable. This way is very effective and the people who do this often go on to become nurses, social workers, carers, therapists etc. They can often be unfulfilled as they have no balance, always giving but not always able to receive back as their identity is only as the giver.

Case Study 3

Moira was a human rights lawyer who only dated what she called losers: alcoholics or unemployed men who had nothing to offer her. When we looked at her past she told me her mother, who was a diplomat's wife, was also an alcoholic who would spend days in bed. Moira would cover up for her mother by disposing of the empty bottles and keeping everyone out of her mother's room at the embassy where they lived so that no one knew. Being able to do this for her mother made her feel very important and valued and it was the only time her mother needed her or gave her any attention. So she learnt at an early age that you are only validated if you look after others and they need to be weak if you are to look after them, hence her need to date weak men so that she could mother them and become indispensable to them. Moira was depressed because her life was unfulfilled and unhappy but as she let go of her identity and security as a carer she was able to find happiness in a relationship based on respect and caring for each other.

Case Study 4

Annette was an exceptionally bright girl who became a nurse to meet her needs for caring, warmth, empathy and love but she had no balance as she gave what she most needed to get back. Although she met her needs for connection and significance through her patients, the patients moved on so her needs were only ever met on a temporary basis. Annette became a comfort eater as she had no balance and no lasting love or meaning in her life outside work. This is quite common, and, though it's not the rule, there is certainly a trend, and in fact studies have shown that up to 80 per cent of nurses can come from dysfunctional families. Annette's cure was to realise that she could receive love as well as give love, by reminding herself that she was lovable and writing out the names of all the people who had loved her and why, and then rereading the list every day so that it became embedded in her. She can now accept she is lovable for who she is, not for what she does, and instead of trying to earn love she is able to accept unconditional love because she knows she is worth it, which in turn increases her confidence.

The third way we try to belong is to become brilliant at something, to prove ourselves to others. For example, at school many children feel a need be brilliant academically or at sport. The drive behind the need to be outstanding is the same as the drive to be a carer in that we become indispensable to the group and they need us as much as we need them, so we feel secure instead of insecure. Back when we lived in tribes the best hunter, the best healer, the best builder was highly valued, so being outstanding at maths, computers or sport as a child and being the best salesman or the best negotiator in the office allows us to feel valued for what we can do because it makes us feel important and needed. However, what we really need is to be valued for who we are. When you say to a child, 'I love you because you are so clever or so smart' what they assume is 'Oh, that's why you love me and if I wasn't maybe you wouldn't.' When you say to someone, 'I love you because you are beautiful', they conclude the same thing: 'That's why you love me but you don't love the real me.' It's why so many beautiful people are insecure: they don't feel loved for themselves, only for their looks. It's also why so many people who are successful appear to lack inner confidence. **When you label someone you limit them**: even so-called positive labels like 'my beautiful girl' or 'my brilliant boy' or 'my little helper' have a downside. We all need to be praised but we need to hear 'I love you because you are you, not because you are beautiful or clever or helpful or funny. That's wonderful too, but I would love you just as much without those things.'

Case Study 5

Steven was a lawyer who was deeply unhappy and suffered chronic depression. Nothing seemed to make him feel good about himself. It was very important that he did well as his family always told him he must be the best and do better than anyone else. If he got 99 per cent in a test they would tell him he should have got 100 per cent; if he didn't get a prize at school they would compare him to the child who did and ask him why he could not do better. His father was a very successful lawyer who Stephen felt he could not live up to. He did not even like law but had been pushed into the family law firm by his father. Because his parents expected perfection from him he expected perfection from himself and as a result he was always unhappy and unsatisfied and never felt he deserved to be pleased or even satisfied with his efforts. When Stephen began to see that his purpose in life was not to re-create his father's life and that the universe would never have created him to be someone who was already here, he left the law and became a golf instructor, something he had always wanted to do but that had been dismissed as a worthless profession by his family. He stopped trying to be perfect and began to enjoy his life rather than making it an ongoing race to achieve perfection to please his family. In doing what he loved, and what he felt he had a longing to do, he stopped being depressed and began to feel happy about himself and his life and he no longer gave his parents the power to make him feel bad about himself or his needs and desires.

Another of my clients, who was a top trader in the City and suffered with manic depression, left to become a teacher and ceased being depressed as the stress of the City was wrong for him. Success is not always about making more money and having lots of status symbols; it's also about having inner peace, liking yourself and being happy doing what inspires you. Statistically, hairdressers are the happiest and most fulfilled out of all professionals because their jobs are creative and because all their needs are met on a day-to-day basis: they have certainty, diversity, connection, significance, they make a difference and they feel appreciated and their jobs are social.

The fourth way of belonging is to be so difficult and belligerent that you don't need to belong, which in turn can take the power away from the people who you depend on, who have the power to reject you or make you feel that you don't fit in. This behaviour is implemented to create security rather than insecurity. Many people who go through life striving to be different are in this category and their behaviour, which is designed to always make them feel in control and secure and therefore not needy and unable to be rejected, can also make them abrasive, difficult, critical and demanding personalities. Bipolar depression is often connected to this type of behaviour. When I was working on a television show I worked with a celebrity who managed to be all four types simultaneously. She was constantly ill on set, requiring a doctor, a chiropractor and occasional hospital visits. She cared for all the other celebrities she was working with and took the role as leader, winning at almost everything by sheer determination. She was also immensely disruptive and difficult and had extreme bipolar disorder and had to be put in rehab before the end of filming. Throughout all of this she was charming and very likeable and as I did therapy with her it was interesting to see that she was from a large family of achievers. Her first sibling had taken the role of the hugely successful one, the next sibling was the very good-looking one, the next was the comedian, the next was always ill and other family members were very disruptive and different so she did not feel there was a role left for her and instead she took a little of all of them. I have worked with other patients who have done the same. This is really hard and ongoing work and the cause of much stress and unhappiness. If you come from a large family and are not the firstborn, or the baby of the family, or the prettiest, or the smartest it can be hard to find your identity. Being sick or being the carer may already be taken by a sibling so being difficult and disruptive is the last option and, if that too is gone, being the comedian may be all that's left. People who have to work so hard to find and maintain an identity can never feel confident and at peace and often become depressed. Children of very famous, very successful or very beautiful parents can often have an especially hard time as their parent took a role and made such a success of it and they can't follow that. It's not uncommon to find a hugely successful parent with one child who followed their success and another who experienced a lot of failure and depression. Kirk Douglas, Paul Newman, Gregory Peck, Burt Bacharach and Mary Tyler Moore all had children who killed themselves because of not feeling good enough and two of Bing Crosby's children committed suicide.

However, you no longer need to belong to your original family and your survival and security are no longer dependent on what they thought of you, so whatever your role as a child was you can leave it in your past and find a better image and identity that suits you and is an asset to you.

Case Study 6

Shirley had suffered depression on and off since her teens. Her mother's favourite phrase was 'I can't cope', so Shirley also feels that she can't cope and has never taken steps to achieve her full potential, always working in jobs that aren't challenging, shunning relationships and not believing in herself or wanting a job that would expect more of her. The depression was useful as it gave her a reason and justification for opting out. Shirley was living a life without risk. Her cure was to emphasise that she is not her mother; she is unique and can cope with anything. By reminding herself of this every day she went on to have a happy relationship and a much more successful career, eventually becoming a CEO. Like many very gifted people, Shirley was not recognised as gifted at school. Very bright children are often bored by conventional teaching so they tune out and underachieve, which then impacts very badly on their confidence and self-esteem as they are labelled as not very bright when this is not true at all; they need to learn in a different way, what is known as outside the box thinking.

If you did not do well at school that does not mean you don't have some outstanding talents. It's never too late to make a success of your life. Some of life's most successful people left school with no qualifications and didn't ever go to university, like Karren Brady, the managing director of Birmingham City Football Club, and Michelle Mone, the founder of Ultimo bras, who left school at fifteen without a career but used her brilliant brain to design a worldwide, bestselling bra based on a very simple idea and became a multimillionaire and Businesswoman of the Year. Philip Green, Alan Sugar, John Humphrys, Richard Branson, A. A. Gill, Michael Parkinson and Vivienne Westwood did not go to university. Bill Gates and Ralph Lauren dropped out of university without a degree to do their own thing. Delia Smith and John Lennon left school without a single O level: John Lennon's school report stated that he was 'on the road to failure'. Gordon Ramsay wanted to join the police or Navy but could not due to lack of O levels. Damien Hirst got an E at A level art yet is now the richest artist in the world today. They may not have had academic qualifications but they did have self-belief, and self-belief can be more of an asset than qualifications.

One of my favourite song lyrics says, 'We do the only dance we have ever known until that dance becomes our own'. You know how it is at a family wedding: people from the Sixties still do their Sixties' moves, while teenagers have their own dance moves that parents and grandparents don't recognise. I have adapted the lyric to, 'We play the only part we have ever known until that part becomes our own'. If you have been depressed for a long time, or were raised by depressed parents, or raised in a dysfunctional family, it can seem impossible to change your part, but it is never too late to get a new and better part, to play a different part in your family dynamics until it too becomes your own and is you. When you play a different part, everyone around you plays a different part too: you can't play tennis with someone who refuses to hit the ball back to you, so when you play the part of someone who is confident and has high self-esteem it will cause your family members to eventually recognise this in you and stop treating you in ways that are inappropriate and outgrown. By incorporating into your behaviour and into your life the techniques in this book you can take on another identity and feel better and happier.

Meeting Your Needs

Scientists and doctors have noted that patients respond very well to positive suggestions. They reason that each of us has two selves – a conscious and a subconscious self. The conscious self that you are aware of has an unreliable memory, whereas the subconscious self has an amazing memory. It registers, without our knowledge, the smallest events and it accepts without reasoning whatever we tell it. If your subconscious believes that you are a confident, secure person then you will be. However, if it has accepted a suggestion that you come from an anxious or depressed family and are helpless to do anything about it, then, notwithstanding the fact that you were born loaded with confidence and self-esteem, you are much more likely to remain insecure, depressed or anxious. That is because these suggestions, which you may not be consciously aware of, form blocks in your mind and are caused by negative beliefs. By changing your belief system as you work your way through this book and repeating your new affirmations as well as regularly playing your audio download, you can and will overcome them. Our subconscious presides over all our actions, whatever they are. Imagination always makes us act, even against our will. It is a rule of the mind that our imagination always beats our willpower; in a battle between willpower and imagination the imagination will always win, without exception. For example, if I asked you to walk a plank of wood placed a few inches off the ground, you would walk along it effortlessly because you would imagine it to be easy. You would see yourself walking across without difficulty. Now, if you to have to imagine walking that same plank of wood when it is placed between two very high buildings, you would feel scared and nervous and you would be very likely to fall off. So why is it that you would not fall off the plank nearer the ground? When the plank was on the ground you believed that you could do it. When the plank was placed between the high buildings you imagined that you could not do it, even if you were offered a lot of money because your imagination sees you falling. In the scenario with the high buildings your will is powerless against your imagination. If you have failed to conquer depression and had no long-term success with medication, your imagination will now see any method failing to work for you. It is the absolute rule of the mind that your imagination will always win. The aim of my programme is to train your imagination so that you will win. Your imagination is like an untamed horse: it is immensely powerful but you have to train it to go where you want it to go. Your imagination and your ability to see yourself recovering from depression while believing that you can become and stay confident and self-assured is powerful and real. Modern science has proved that the way you think can physically change your life. Changing your thinking can and does change your life and it can and does end depression.

I know you don't just want to hear this. To believe it you need to see it and experience it for yourself. The following test will do that for you. Many of my clients find this very useful because it gives them absolute proof that our thoughts affect our body. Once you have that proof you can never again say, 'I can't help it, it's just the way I am.' The truth is it's the way you think, not the way you are, and the following test will really change your thinking, which in turn will change your body.

Exercise 1

I am hopeless and depressed v. I am confident and capable

You need someone to help you do this. Stand up with your feet slightly apart and your arms by your side. Now think of the most negative words or beliefs you use about yourself in relation to confidence or depression. Repeat these words out loud ten times or just think them silently, ten times. An example could be:

I am hopeless and inadequate' or

'I can't talk to people'

'I am depressed'

'I am shy' or *'I am not good enough'*

Now, thinking these thoughts, get your helper to push you on your shoulders or chest so that you are being pushed backwards. Don't worry: you won't fall, you may step back a little but you won't fall over.

You will find that as you think negative thoughts you lose your strength and you can easily be pushed off balance.

Amazing, isn't it? When you think those negative thoughts you are losing all your strength and becoming weak; you are weaker while thinking those thoughts.

This is even more proof of the amazing powers of the mind.

This time, think of some positive words or beliefs to use about yourself, repeat them silently or out loud ten times or repeat any of the suggestions below ten times:

'I am supremely confident and self-assured'
'I am confident'
'I have a totally different attitude to life'
'People like me'
'I am well and happy'

Now, thinking these thoughts have your helper repeat the pushing and you will find that you stay anchored and rooted to the ground. You will be strong enough to resist the pushing. Isn't it great to see that, as you think positive thoughts, you become physically stronger and it is easy for you to resist the pushing?

I mentioned earlier that every thought you have creates a physical reaction in the body and you have just proved it to yourself.

Where a thought goes energy goes with it, so, you see, changing your thinking and using different language really does change your body.

Most people are fascinated by this testing and since it's a fun thing to do I recommend you spend some time experimenting with it.

1. Repeating all the negative thoughts and beliefs you had.
2. Using all the negative words you had been using before realising the power of language.
3. Testing your strength.
4. Replacing these negative beliefs with positive, constructive beliefs.
5. Testing your strength again and seeing the difference.

You can do this with so many beliefs about your confidence, self-esteem, habits, abilities and relationships – in fact anything at all.

Remember, these beliefs only exist in your imagination and you are free to change your thinking and your language as soon as you become aware of how limiting and destructive your language and beliefs are.

While the mind does run the body it is your mind and you are able to direct it, to change it and to influence positive changes in yourself. Changing your language and your beliefs is one of the quickest ways to do this.

- Your thoughts are yours to change.
- Your mind is yours to direct.
- Your beliefs about your confidence and self-esteem are absolutely yours to change.

I want you to spend at least five minutes really doing this next exercise and giving it 100 per cent.

Ask yourself what it is costing you to live below your potential? What will it go on costing you? What price are you paying when you hold yourself back? Are you prepared to pay that price? What are you missing out on?

I want you to really think about your answers and write them down. Make a list of what it is costing you. Write out what you feel you are missing out on.

Keep going until you have exhausted your answers and then read through your list again and decide if you are prepared to pay that price; or are you ready for a new mindset, one that will work for you rather than against you?

Once you've finished your list, I want you to focus on the next exercise. Don't just read it and move on. You must DO it. This is not just a book for you to read, it's a book for you to use. It's a programme rather than a book and the results you will get from this programme will come about as a result of you processing the information and doing the exercises. Fully participating in them forms part of that process. So for real results, read through the next paragraph, memorise it and then go back and do it and do it fully. Give it 100 per cent and that's what you will get back.

This last exercise is designed to safely change the neural pathways in your brain, which will change your inner confidence. Please take the time to do it rather than just reading it as the effects are very powerful and a key part of this programme. Again, read through and memorise the next exercise, then do it.

Exercise 2

Close your eyes and imagine you are now at your best. I want you to see what you could buy that could give you the same feeling as being your best. Could you find a car, a house, a boat, an outfit, a new state-of-the-art gizmo, some gourmet food? After a while you will notice there is nothing, no items that can ever give you that feeling. Even if you could find some purchase that would make you feel good it would not last. You get used to purchases. When I got my first sports car no one was allowed to eat in it. I kept a towel on the floor to keep it immaculate and then I got used to it and eventually it became just a car. New clothes, shoes and carpets make us feel good for a brief period of time and then we have to move on to more stuff, to keep filling the emptiness inside. Advertisers know this and constantly pitch the latest must have but when you truly like yourself and feel good about yourself you don't need so much stuff. It also helps to work out how long you feel good for after acquiring stuff and how long you feel good for when you like yourself. Remember everything you think you want is because of how you think it will make you feel. You can get the feeling without needing the purchases.

As I have already said, one of the definitions of madness is doing the same thing over and over again while expecting a different result. You are ready to do and think differently and you will get different results, permanently.

Now go ahead and really do the exercise so you can discover this for yourself. *Imagine* yourself in detail really liking yourself, how you'd look and feel and how people would see you.

STEP 10

'If you want the present to be different from the past, study the past' – Baruch Spinoza, 1632–77, Dutch philosopher

Ten Ways to Feel Good About Yourself

Even though some of these steps may be condensed and repeated from previous chapters your mind learns by repetition. Repetition is the mother of all skills and this chapter is a summary of everything you have learnt and need in order to have a confident life and a confident future.

1. LIKE YOURSELF. OTHER PEOPLE WILL LIKE YOU TO THE DEGREE THAT YOU LIKE YOURSELF.

We can all find something to like about ourselves. What you look like is just the wrapping. Think of all the compliments you have ever been given and remember them. The more you like yourself the more other people will like you and feel reassured around you. The minute you like yourself your sense of self-worth and self-esteem goes up and as you increase your own sense of self-worth everyone around you increases their sense of your worth too. We live in a world where we believe that continually improving ourselves is the key to happiness. That is not strictly correct. Accepting ourselves is the key to happiness and confidence. There is a cosmetic surgery clinic called Transform and its message is that when you transform your body you will be happy. A younger face or a smaller nose will make you happy and confident and yet I have worked with many cosmetic surgeons who send me clients that worry them because they keep coming back for more and more surgery. The nose is still not quite right or now they want liposuction or a tummy tuck as well. Transformation begins when you like yourself and can see all the good things about yourself. You don't transform by working out or having liposuction; you transform by seeing all the good things about you and when you see them everyone else will see them too. That does not mean that you should not make the best of yourself but it does mean that you recognise that there is no destination called confidence or happiness that you will arrive at one day. Happiness and confidence are the journey. You will meet your need for **significance** by liking yourself.

2. DON'T TRY TO BE PERFECT.

You are entering a race that you can't win; you can't even finish as the finishing line always moves beyond your reach. Your race to reach perfection is an optical illusion; it's a mirage. People who seek and appear to need perfection have been proved to be the unhappiest and most unsatisfied people in the world. You will meet your need for **acceptance** when you stop trying to be perfect.

3. FIND OUT WHAT YOU LOVE TO DO AND DO IT.

We all have a gift and our gifts lie right behind and are directly connected to what we love doing and what we loved doing between the ages of seven and fourteen. When we do what we love we shine and understand why we are on the planet. We recognise the genius in ourselves and we do all have it. You were not put here just to find love. We are here to understand our talents and use them. What did you love to do when you were a kid?

What do you love doing now? You can only truly be successful when you do something you love. You will meet your need for **contribution** when you do what you love.

4. SET YOURSELF GOALS AND MOVE TOWARDS THEIR ACHIEVEMENT.

Our brains are natural goal-seeking mechanisms. With goals we have purpose and direction. Without them we drift and flounder. Authentic happiness comes from setting yourself goals and moving towards their accomplishment. Happiness is not only the goal destination, it's the goal journey. We are just as happy moving towards our goals as when achieving them. That's why so many people who have achieved a goal go on to achieve another one. You will meet your need for **growth** when you move towards and reach your goals.

5i. BE ALTRUISTIC.

Scientists have found that doing something nice for others, no matter how small, makes us feel better and for longer than buying clothes or shoes or comfort eating. Practise spontaneous acts of generosity and kindness. If you're stuck in a traffic queue and someone wants to join the line, let them in. You'll feel good about yourself, and you'll reach where you were going in almost the same length of time, except you'll be significantly less stressed and better able to cope with what you're doing when you get there. At the supermarket if someone does not have enough money at the till give it to them. I have had so many BIG successes and wonderful moments in my life to remember but what I also remember are little things like someone at the queue making up my money when I was short and doing the same thing for other people who were short of money at the checkout. I also remember a man's face at a tube station when I gave him his fare; he was looking so distressed as he didn't have enough money, and when I gave him the money he looked as if he had just won the lottery and his happiness gave me back so much more than the few pounds I gave him. The thing I remember the most is a small boy whose family had no money coming to our house when I was about fourteen to collect a bike my dad had promised him. Dad had found it abandoned at his school and was working in the garage restoring it so this little boy would have a bike. As I took him to the garage he said to me, 'Your dad is so kind. Is he Jesus?' My dad showed me that life is about making a difference. He was always helping people and I am so glad I learnt from him. You will meet your need for **connection** when you do this.

5ii. PRAISE MORE AND CRITICISE LESS (ESPECIALLY YOURSELF).

Praise boosts our self-esteem and criticism withers it. Superior people praise others and people who dislike themselves are very critical of others. They express outwardly their own feelings of discontent. When you praise someone you also benefit as when we give a compliment we get something back. You can always find something nice to say to someone. When you boost someone else's self-esteem you boost your own. Try telling the supermarket cashier that she has lovely nails or hair, or you love her perfume, and you will both benefit. Scientists have shown that doing or saying something nice to others gives us longer lasting pleasure than chocolate. Give lots of compliments, including to yourself. It's easy to find something nice to say to someone but it has to be sincere. You can tell anyone that they are doing a great job and you can give yourself a compliment all the time. Don't hold back: you deserve compliments and if you are not getting enough give them to yourself – simple things like 'I did a great job', 'I look lovely', 'I'm a good person', 'I like myself'. You will meet your need for **certainty** by complimenting yourself and others. You are meeting your need to be free from **rejection** every time you do this.

The key to inner happiness is an ability to express hurt and a willingness to do it as close to the event that hurt you as possible. All anger is hurt that has not been expressed so get into the excellent habit of saying, 'My feelings were hurt when you forgot my birthday, cancelled lunch, didn't show up' rather than saying, 'You made me mad when you forgot my birthday. I was really angry when you didn't show up.' Even worse is keeping those feeling in. They have to find an outlet somewhere and unexpressed hurt can make you tense, anxious and ill. If you can't tell someone like a boss or relative that they have hurt you, say it out loud in private instead and it will still have a better effect on your self-esteem than keeping it inside. You will meet your need for **inner peace** by expressing your hurt.

Even when things are going wrong you can still think, 'What is good about this?' It sounds crazy, I know, but it works and you can find out what's good about anything if you look. What's good about being stuck in traffic? You have a car. What's good about the queue in Tesco? You live in a country with an abundance of food and you have enough money to buy it. Whatever your problem is, it is another person's absolute fantasy dream come true. They would love to have a job that's stressful, a partner who is messy, a child who is expensive, a baby who keeps them up at night or a house that needs constant upkeep, a dishwasher that no one else in the family bothers to empty. By focusing on all the things that are great you focus on what you have instead of what you don't have. It also helps to think about what you would have given ten years ago to have the problem you have now. For example, when I drove my daughter to school each day I was thinking negatively and hating the journey. I was using really negative words like, 'Because of road works the road was reduced to one lane for what seemed like an *eternity* and the drive, which already took *forever*, became *horrendous*' until one day, sitting in my car, in the rain, waiting for the traffic to move, I looked at a woman standing at the bus stop with her son and realised how lucky I was. I had a car, I was driving my daughter to a fantastic school that I was lucky enough to choose and I had the time to drive her to school. When I was in the supermarket queue to pay for my shopping and the person in front was giving new meaning to the word slow, I made myself do the same thing and say, 'How lucky am I to be in this shop with money to buy whatever food I choose, to take home to the dinner party I am having for people that I love who love me.' I probably sound nauseatingly glib about it but I don't like food shopping and I don't always like cooking and moments before I was doing the 'God I hate shopping, this all takes so much time, I have to buy it, pack it, put it the car, drive home, unpack it, prepare it and then clean up' until I reminded myself why I was giving a dinner party.

I was shamed into thinking this way when I took my Croatian au pair into Sainsbury's with me and she burst into tears at the sight of so much abundant food as at that time (in 1994) her family had no access to food and no money to buy it and she was sending parcels of packet soup home to them. She taught me to focus on how lucky I am. Hell is not being in Tesco, the queues in Asda are not a nightmare. Again, your problem is someone else's fantasy dream come true. You will meet your need for **gratitude** and **appreciation** by doing this.

8. USE THE WORDS 'I AM CHOOSING TO OR CHOOSING NOT TO'.

Studies have shown that very successful people never say 'I can't or I can'; they say 'I am choosing to or choosing not to'. By speaking in this manner they feel in control of themselves and their destiny. It is not possible to feel truly good about ourselves unless we feel that we can shape and influence the direction of change going on in our lives. Just changing the words you use can have a dramatic change on your feelings. You will meet your need for **certainty** as you do this.

9. EAT SOME SEROTONIN-BOOSTING FOODS EVERY DAY.

Serotonin is a feel-good hormone and many binge eaters, depressives and alcoholics lack serotonin. The biggest boosters of serotonin are coriander, bananas, eggs, turkey, dates, pears, avocados and very dark chocolate. Taking vitamin B complex and vitamin B6 will also increase serotonin.

10i. BE TACTILE: TOUCH SOMEONE EVERY DAY.

Touching others releases oxytocin, the love hormone. Looking into the eyes of someone you love also releases oxytocin. Even if you don't have a partner to love and touch, hugging friends and children or stroking pets has a similar effect. People love people who are warm and empathetic so don't hold back. Just touching someone on the arm as you talk to them makes an impact and causes them to remember you and like you more. You will meet your need for **connection** through touch.

Sex improves our happiness levels as we experience a huge surge of the calming love hormone oxytocin. Just getting close to your partner and staring into their eyes for five minutes releases oxytocin. After sex the happiness hormone serotonin is released. This can elevate our mood for the rest of the day. Recent studies have shown that orgasm is vital to a healthy immune system. Women who reach orgasm regularly survive breast cancer more than those who don't. Orgasm boosts NK (natural killer) cells and T cells, it makes you look and feel younger too. DIY orgasms have the same effect. Prostaglandin is a mood-elevating hormone released in semen and absorbed in women that makes women happy. Obviously, only have unprotected sex with a regular partner. You will meet your need for **diversity** doing this.

Peer Pressure: to Sum it All Up

- Do something nice for someone else every day.
- Do something nice for yourself every day.
- Take a risk every day including expressing your feelings.
- Give a compliment daily and also compliment yourself.
- Be grateful and appreciative (an attitude to gratitude).
- Talk to yourself in a more confident way.
- STOP all negative self-criticism for good.
- Walk and move like a confident person.
- Visualise regularly and keep big, confident pictures in your head.
- Remember you are lovable and you are ENOUGH.
- Become a natural goal setter.
- Only use confident, positive language.

As you embrace everything in this book you will change.

When this happens watch out because you will have new symptoms including but not limited to:

- Being spontaneous instead of fearful anxious or self-conscious.
- Living in the moment and enjoying the moment.
- Loss of interest in judging or criticising others or yourself.
- Loss of interest in arguing or worrying or proving that you were right.
- Feelings of appreciation, contentment, gratitude and connectedness.
- Letting things happen with no need to be in control.
- Feeling warm and loving to others and noticing and letting them be warm and loving to you.
- Uncontrollable urges to smile laugh and let others in.
- Truly liking yourself and feeling good about who you are and why you are here.

Be aware: these are very serious symptoms likely to baffle and confuse people around you who may resist your changes initially and be irked by your happiness, while others will love you more for it and radiate towards you because of it.

I have to end with a quote that is so relevant. Barack Obama said, 'Change will not come if we wait for some other person or some other time. We are the ones we have been waiting for, we are the change that we seek.' But this is not an ending; it's a new beginning. You have learnt so much, starting by changing your attitude and then your language, before choosing to be confident. You have taken lots of small steps that get big results and you are finally able to get the confidence and self-esteem you were meant to have by making mental changes and taking actions that bring results that make it worth it. You have learnt to reactivate innate confidence and know that continuously visualising yourself as confident and self-assured is not some new age hocus-pocus but a science that really works. You know how to visualise your progress for lasting success and how to set goals and make them work for you.

You have learnt how to communicate and made changes that are physical and mental, so you have changed from the inside as well as on the outside. As a grand finale, you know how to be confident in your career and your relationships and I know that you can do it. The ten new ways to stay confident will help remind you how to continuously act and react like a naturally confident person, which is what you will become and remain. Being confident does not mean you will never meet challenges; it means you will always bounce right back and you have the different scripts in Step 6 to use whenever you need them. You won't ever give up just because you have had a bad day. After all, you wouldn't go on to empty out your bank account just because you have overspent, would you? Being naturally confident and self-assured is how you are going to be almost all the time. The thing I love the most about my programme is that you don't have to do all of it all the time for it to work. As long as you do most of it most of the time it will work.

It's essential that you have not only read this book from cover to cover but that you have done all the exercise required (if you have skipped any of them please go back and do them right now, not for me but for you). I designed these exercises so that you can be confident, so please do them. From the beginning to the end of this book you have been absorbing powerful, workable solutions to being confident and self-assured and radiating high self-esteem. You cannot adhere to this programme without seeing and feeling the benefits. As long as you use this book the way it was meant to be used you will have Ultimate Confidence.

A Day in the Life of the New Confident You

Be confident, be happy and know that you are always enough. Express your hurt when it occurs, stop all negative self-criticism and really like yourself for who you are and know that you are unique, you matter, you are here for a reason with something valuable to contribute. If you do that and incorporate the techniques in this book you will always have Ultimate Confidence. And remember, when you make yourself a better person you help to make the world a better place.

If you slip up, go back to the appropriate chapter; if you are still hard on yourself reread the chapter on changing your language. Keep on working on your goals and put the information into practice. If other people resist the new, confident you, reread Step 7 on relationship communication and, remember, this is all about you; you don't need to convert anyone (unless, of course, they want you to, in which case please do) and neither can anyone convert you back to those old bad habits unless you let them, and you are never going to do that. If any particular chapter in this programme caused you to really resonate with something I said then go back and read that chapter again. Print out some of the sayings if they were particularly helpful and remember them.

Remember you have been through a hypnotic process and you have worked hard to make powerful and lasting changes. They won't undo themselves and if you are at all worried that they will remember you have an additional special tool, your audio download (see Contents page). Repetition is called the mother of all skills. Remember that I told you that repeating actions creates a neural pathway to the brain that is reinforced with every repetition. When you play this audio download and see yourself as confident and self-assured you are sending messages to your subconscious mind that further help you to become this way. You will be continuously reinforcing all the good changes you are making until they stick and you are rewired to respond to any and every situation with increased confidence.

Every time you play it you are re-enforcing your mind and replacing old, negative suggestions with powerful, positive ones. As you play the audio download the image of you at your best, radiating a natural, reassuring confidence will become more real and more attainable each time you hear it. The audio download is going to help you so much. It will have a powerful, permanent and all-pervasive impact on your self-image, your confidence and your beliefs, so play it every day without a break for twenty-one days (remember those neural pathways changing after twenty-one days) and then continue to play it regularly until the words become deeply embedded and encoded into your subconscious mind.

I hope you have enjoyed this journey to be confident, to truly like yourself without having to try too hard. The destination is fantastic. It's you feeling the way you were meant to feel but the journey is quite an accomplishment too. Thank you so much for taking it with me. Please keep in touch with me and let me know your progress. You can email me for advice on www.marisapeer.com or info@marisapeer.com. I hope to meet you one day at one of my seminars.

Here's looking at (the new confident) you.
Love from,

Marisa Peer

Appendix

p. 23 'This can then produce NK killer cells . . .' Martin L. Rossman, *Guided Imagery for Self-healing* (California, New World Library), 2000

p. 32 'The pioneer of this . . .' Marva Collins with Civia Tamarkin, *Marva Collins' Way* (USA, Penguin group) 1990; Marva Collins, *Ordinary Children, Extraordinary Teachers* (USA, Hampton Roads Publishing) 2003; P. Kamara Sekou Collins, *The School That Cared: A Story of the Marva Collins Preparatory School of Cincinnati* (USA, University Press of America) 2003; www.marvacollins.com

p. 37 'A recent experiment looked at waitresses and waiters . . .', Nicolas Guéguen and Céline Jacob, *The Effect of Tactile Stimulation on the Purchasing Behaviour of Consumers: An Experimental Study in a Natural Setting, International Journal of Management*, Mar 2006. http://findarticles.com/p/articles/mi_qa5440/is_200603/ai_n21388596/pg_2

p. 38 'The human brain produces approximately 50,000, thoughts a day . . .' *Science Daily* (December 18, 2006). http://www.sciencedaily.com.

p. 47 'I read a story about a man . . .' Brian Tracy, *Goals! How to Get Everything You Want – Faster Than You Ever Thought Possible* (Berrett-Koehler), 2001. Reprinted with permission of the publisher. From *Goals*, copyright© (2001) by Brian Tracy, Berrett-Koehler Publishers, Inc., Francisco, CA. All rights reserved. www.bkconnection.com

p. 55 'Marilyn Monroe . . .' Mike Evans, *The Marilyn Handbook* (MQ Publications), 2004

p. 57 'Patti Boyd said that . . .' Patti Boyd, *Wonderful Today* (UK, Headline Review), 2008

p. 96 'In Mark McCormack's book . . .' Mark McCormack, *What They Don't Teach You at Harvard Business School* (UK, Bantam), 1986

p. 97 'Louis Pasteur said . . .' John Cook, Steve Deger and Leslie Ann Gibson, *The Book of Positive Quotations* (USA, Fairview Press), 2007

p. 97 'Brian Tracy states that . . .' Brian Tracy, *Goals! How to Get Everything You Want – Faster Than You Ever Thought Possible*

p. 106 'The Pareto principle proves that . . .' www.theparetoprinciple.com

p. 107 'Studies show that . . .' Education Policy Analysis Archives, College of Education, University of South Florida

p. 109 'Any goal of significance . . .' www.quotations.com

p. 110 'Someone once told Michael Jordan . . .' www.quotations.com

p. 111 'Failures will put off . . .' Brian Tracy, *The Psychology of Achievement* (Nightingale Conant), 1984

p. 116 '"Carefully watch your thoughts . . ."' www.trans4mind.com

p. 152 'Within a year of marriage . . .' World Values Survey, The Pew Research Center, 2007

p. 180 'Ideas that have a strong emotional content . . .' Gil Boyne, *Transforming Therapy* (USA, Westwood Publishing Co)

p. 204 'At Bellevue Psychiatric Hospital . . .' Norman Cousins, *Anatomy of an Illness* (USA, Bantam), 1991

p. 213 'Statistically, hairdressers are the happiest . . .' Department of Trade and Industry survey 2004 and 2006. The *Journal of Psychological Science* found that happy people spent the least time alone and the most time socialising with others.